2969
GM.MTQ/LeV

D1765372

THIS BOOK BELONGS TO:
Kostoris Library
Christie Hospital NHS Trust
Manchester
M20 4BX
Phone: 0161 446 3452

2969
GM.MTQ/LeV

Clinical Lymphatic Mapping in Gynecologic Cancers

DEDICATION

To my parents, Hedi Basch Levenback and Robert Levenback, whose courage and determination inspire me. To my wife, Ginny, whose love and support bring joy to my life. To my sons, Sam and Ben, who give me hope for the future.

Charles Levenback

To my parents, Biny Van der Zee-Muntingh and Martin van der Zee, for their love and long-lasting support. To my wife, Joukje van der Naalt and my children, Wierd, Heleen and Hannah, for bringing so much joyful distraction into my life.

Ate G.J. van der Zee

To my wife, Fay, whose love, insight and daily selfless sacrifice strengthen and inspire me. To my children, Jay, Christina, Kay, Joe and Mary who bring true color and happiness to my life. To my patients whose charity of self makes this endeavor possible.

Robert L. Coleman

Clinical Lymphatic Mapping in Gynecologic Cancers

Edited by

Charles Levenback M.D.
University of Texas M.D. Anderson Cancer Center
Houston
Texas
USA

Ate G.J. van der Zee M.D. Ph.D.
University Hospital
Groningen
The Netherlands

Robert L. Coleman M.D.
University of Texas Southwestern Medical Center
Dallas
Texas
USA

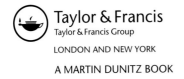
Taylor & Francis
Taylor & Francis Group

LONDON AND NEW YORK

A MARTIN DUNITZ BOOK

© 2004 Taylor & Francis, an imprint of the Taylor & Francis Group

First published in the United Kingdom in 2004
by Taylor & Francis, an imprint of the Taylor & Francis Group, 11 New Fetter Lane, London EC4P 4EE

Tel.:   +44 (0) 20 7583 9855
Fax.:   +44 (0) 20 7842 2298
E-mail: info@dunitz.co.uk
Website: http://www.dunitz.co.uk

All rights reserved. No part of this publication may be reproduced, stored in a retrieval system, or transmitted, in any form or by any means, electronic, mechanical, photocopying, recording, or otherwise, without the prior permission of the publisher or in accordance with the provisions of the Copyright, Designs and Patents Act 1988 or under the terms of any licence permitting limited copying issued by the Copyright Licensing Agency, 90 Tottenham Court Road, London W1P 0LP.

Although every effort has been made to ensure that all owners of copyright material have been acknowledged in this publication, we would be glad to acknowledge in subsequent reprints or editions any omissions brought to our attention.

The Author has asserted his right under the Copyright, Designs and Patents Act 1988 to be identified as the Author of this Work.

Although every effort has been made to ensure that drug doses and other information are presented accurately in this publication, the ultimate responsibility rests with the prescribing physician. Neither the publishers nor the authors can be held responsible for errors or for any consequences arising from the use of information contained herein. For detailed prescribing information or instructions on the use of any product or procedure discussed herein, please consult the prescribing information or instructional material issued by the manufacturer.

A CIP record for this book is available from the British Library.

Library of Congress Cataloging-in-Publication Data

Data available on application

ISBN 1 84184 276 1

Distributed in North and South America by
Taylor & Francis
2000 NW Corporate Blvd
Boca Raton, FL 33431, USA

Within Continental USA
Tel: 800 272 7737; Fax: 800 374 3401
Outside Continental USA
Tel: 561 994 0555; Fax: 561 361 6018
E-mail: orders@crcpress.com

Distributed in the rest of the world by
Thomson Publishing Services
Cheriton House
North Way
Andover, Hampshire SP10 5BE, UK
Tel.:   +44 (0)1264 332424
E-mail: salesorder.tandf@thomsonpublishingservices.co.uk

Production editor: Julian Evans

Composition by J&L Composition, Filey, North Yorkshire, UK

Printed and bound in Spain by Grafos SA

CONTENTS

Contributors vi

Preface vii

1 THE HISTORY OF LYMPHATIC MAPPING:
A GYNECOLOGIC PERSPECTIVE 1
Charles Levenback

2 LYMPHATIC ANATOMY 15

   a Microanatomy and physiology of the human lymphatic system
    Charles Levenback

   b Lymphatics of the vulva
    Robert L. Coleman

   c Lymphatics of the cervix
    Robert L. Coleman

   d Lymphatics of the corpus uteri
    Ate G.J. van der Zee

   e Lymphatics of the ovary
    Ate G.J. van der Zee

   f Lymphatic anatomy of the breast and axilla
    James V. Florica

3 MODALITIES OF DETECTION OF SENTINEL NODES IN
LYMPHATIC MAPPING 67
Pedro T. Ramirez and Charles Levenback

4 ULTRASTAGING OF THE SENTINEL NODE 85
Paul J. van Diest and Ate G.J. van der Zee

5 SENTINEL LYMPH NODE PROCEDURE IN VULVAR CANCER 101
JA de Hullu and Ate G.J. van der Zee

6 SENTINEL LYMPH NODE MAPPING IN CERVIX CANCER 125
Robert L. Coleman and Charles Levenback

7 SENTINEL LYMPH NODE MAPPING IN BREAST CANCER 147
Mary L. Gemignani

8 SENTINEL LYMPH NODE MAPPING IN ENDOMETRIAL CANCER 171
Charles Levenback

9 DIFFUSION OF INNOVATION AND CLINICAL TRIAL DESIGN IN
LYMPHATIC MAPPING 179
Charles Levenback

Index 191

CONTRIBUTORS

Robert L. Coleman M.D.
University of Texas Southwestern Medical Center
Dallas
Texas
USA

Paul J. van Diest M.D. Ph.D.
Department of Pathology
University Medical Center Utrecht
Utrecht
The Netherlands

James V. Florica M.D.
University of South Florida
Tampa
Florida
USA

Mary L. Gemignani M.D.
Memorial Sloan-Kettering Cancer Center
New York
New York
USA

JA de Hullu M.D. Ph.D.
University Hospital
Groningen
The Netherlands

Charles Levenback M.D.
M.D. Anderson Cancer Center
Houston
Texas
USA

Pedro T. Ramirez M.D.
M.D. Anderson Cancer Center
Houston
Texas
USA

Ate G.J. van der Zee M.D. Ph.D.
University Hospital
Groningen
The Netherlands

PREFACE

It is with a great sense of accomplishment that we present the first comprehensive text of lymphatic mapping in gynecologic cancers. The catalyst for this book was a postgraduate course we taught at the annual meetings of the Society of Gynecologic Oncologists, and the many requests from attendees from around the world for resources and references regarding mapping. We were often asked if there was a single resource for a gynecologic oncologist interested in lymphatic mapping. Since there was none, we set out to fill this gap.

In our initial discussions of the contents of the book, we identified the importance of a historical perspective, an understanding of the associated modalities (pathology and diagnostic imaging), as well as a disease site-specific review of the literature and step-by-step descriptions of how to identify sentinel nodes. During these discussions, we found the work of the anatomists of the 19th and 20th centuries of particular relevance and importance. This body of literature was exhaustively reviewed and illustrated by Albert Plentl and Emanuel Friedman in their book *Lymphatics of the Female Genital Tract*. Although it had been long out of print, we still found ourselves turning to decades-old copies of this volume. The more we learned about mapping, the more we wanted to know about the lymphatic anatomy of the groin and pelvis. This included many of the anatomic variations that we encountered in the operating room, observing blue dye in lymphatic channels and lymph nodes. We decided that a full appreciation of lymphatic mapping is predicated on a firm understanding of the complexity and nuances of lymphatic anatomy and we have aimed to provide this to our readers.

We strongly believe that lymphatic mapping procedures will result in better outcomes for patients, due to improved detection of metastatic disease and reduced surgical morbidity. We also realize that the evidence to substantially change some of our standard operative management is still lacking. We have presented our interpretation of the data. However, we encourage our readers to critically analyze the data for themselves, and maintain a healthy degree of skepticism in evaluating the procedures described in these pages.

We are grateful to the many mentors and colleagues in our professional lives who have supported our careers in general and this project specifically. We wish to acknowledge the energy and creativity of the many gynecologic oncologists who share the mission of reducing the burden of cancer on the women of the world. We sincerely hope that this book contributes to that mission.

Charles Levenback
Ate G.J. van der Zee
Robert L. Coleman

1 HISTORY OF LYMPHATIC MAPPING: A GYNECOLOGIC PERSPECTIVE

Charles Levenback

INTRODUCTION

In the new millennium, it is commonly believed that the answers to cancer questions will result from innovations in molecular biology that are brought from the bench to the bedside through the work of translational researchers. However, the story of the development of lymphatic mapping serves as a reminder to us that, even now, some advances in cancer care still come from the more traditional routes of careful study of anatomy, clinical observation, and literature research.

The history of the development of lymphatic mapping is also a humbling lesson in how important innovations in medicine can diffuse slowly. The term 'sentinel node' was first used in 1960,[1] yet even today the full potential of this concept has not been realized. Initial reports of success with the sentinel node concept were largely ignored or misinterpreted. Old ideas can be difficult to abandon, and new ideas are not always what they appear.

The relative infrequency of gynecologic tumors is an additional impediment to development of lymphatic mapping in our specialty. Fortunately, we can learn a lot from the experience of others in treating more common diseases. The purpose of this chapter is to introduce the concept of the lymphatic mapping and sentinel lymph node biopsy with a special emphasis on how the development of lymphatic mapping intertwined with surgical advances in gynecologic oncology. Subsequent chapters will review the lymphatic anatomy of the female lower genital tract and breast and the current state of knowledge regarding lymphatic mapping for tumors at these sites.

CADAVER STUDIES OF LYMPHATIC ANATOMY

Early anatomists learned about lymphatic anatomy from cadavers. This work was complicated by the fact that lymphatic channels are difficult to see and very fragile, and by the fact that tissue had to be extensively putrefied or fixed to be studied. Painstaking dissections led to the production of remarkable drawings of lymphatic anatomy. These illustrations were frequently reproduced by subsequent investigators with small improvements (Figures 1.1 and 1.2). Anatomists developed a variety of aids to help visualize the lymphatic channels, including a number of mercurial compounds that, when injected into various soft tissues, canalized the lymphatics. This technique most likely contributed to the depictions of lymphatic anatomy that erroneously show vulvar lymphatics crossing the labial-crural fold, best represented by Sappey's illustration (Figure 1.3). In the early twentieth century, the French gynecologists Leveuf and Godard[2] studied the lymphatic anatomy of the cervix using injection of Gerotti blue into the cervices of neonatal cadavers. They found that the dye drained in a highly reproducible way to a lymph node usually found in the obturator space or close to the iliac vessels. They named this the 'principal' lymph node (Figure 1.4).

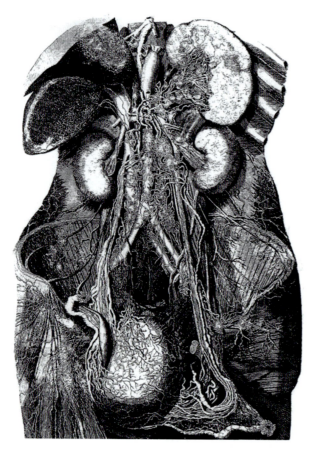

Figure 1.1 Lymphatics of the abdomen and pelvis (1787) by P. Mascagni (reproduced from Plentl and Friedman, *Lymphatics of Female Genital Tract*)[4] with permission from Elsevier.

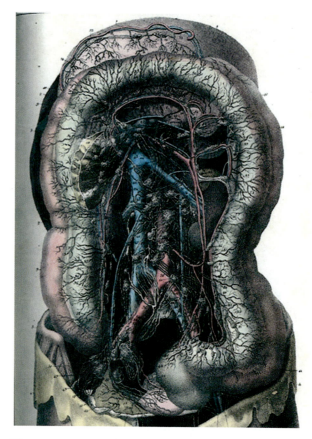

Figure 1.2 Lymphatics of the abdomen and pelvis (from a nineteenth-century French textbook).

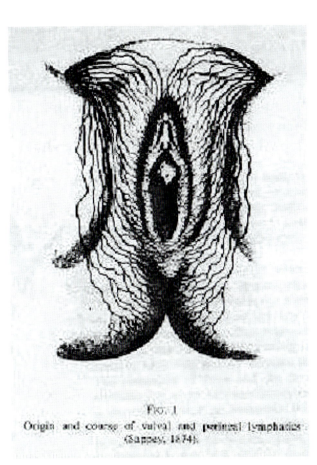

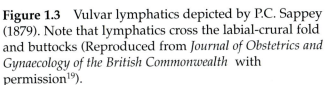

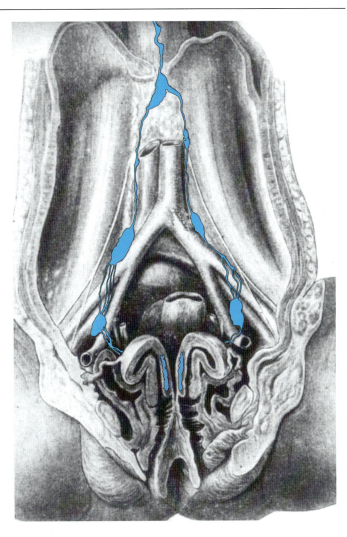

Figure 1.3 Vulvar lymphatics depicted by P.C. Sappey (1879). Note that lymphatics cross the labial-crural fold and buttocks (Reproduced from *Journal of Obstetrics and Gynaecology of the British Commonwealth* with permission[19]).

Figure 1.4 Leveuf and Godard's[2] description (1923) of lymphatic drainage of the cervix (courtesy Dr Daniel Dargent).

HALSTED MODEL FOR SURGICAL MANAGEMENT OF SOLID TUMORS

The great anatomist of the second century, Galen, believed that cancer was a local process resulting from a systemic disease of bodily fluids and humors. In the West, this concept was not challenged until the seventeenth century, when Valsalva proposed that cancer spread from primary tumors to lymph nodes.[3] This understanding of cancer and the metastatic process ultimately led to the Halstedian model for surgical management of solid tumors. In this model, the primary tumor, the primary regional lymph nodes, and the second-echelon regional nodes, as well as all of the intervening lymphatic channels—including the fine cutaneous lymphatics—were resected en bloc (Figure 1.5). This approach was integrated into the treatment of gynecologic cancers by several gynecologic surgeons working in multiple sites on the European continent. Rupprecht, Basset, Stoeckel, and Bucura are credited with simultaneous descriptions in 1912 of what we now refer to as radical vulvectomy and bilateral inguinal femoral lymphadenectomy.[4] The next generation of gynecologic cancer surgeons, including Twombly,[5] Taussig,[6] and Way,[7] championed radical vulvectomy and bilateral inguinal femoral lymphadenectomy, with only minor revisions for patients with vulvar cancer, because of the dramatic improvement in survival compared with less radical or nonsurgical treatments. Stanley Way summarized the surgical philosophy of the day in 1951 when he stated, 'The most important steps in the operation are undoubtedly the *very wide* removal of the vulva and the resection of the lymph nodes, certainly as far as the node of Cloquet'[8] (Figure 1.6). Way added that the morbidity and mortality of the procedure were justified and that the operation 'represents the final achievement of surgery in this disease'. Within a generation, however, the radicality of surgical treatment of the vulva would be diminishing, and, today, no indications remain for radical vulvectomy and bilateral inguinal femoral lymphadenectomy for the primary treatment of vulvar cancer.

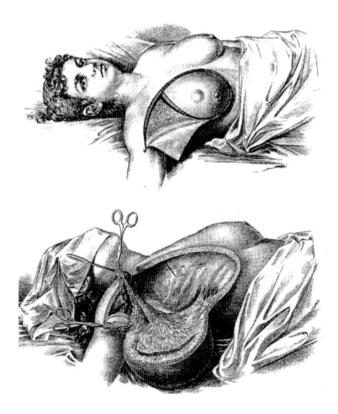

Figure 1.5 The noted surgeon William Halsted based his surgical approach to breast cancer on the concept that the primary tumor was connected to the regional lymph nodes by a network of lymphatic channels in the skin and subcutaneous tissues that had to be resected 'en bloc' ensure resection of lymph node and in transit metastases. This approach was adopted in other disease sites including the vulva. (Reproduced from Rutkow IM, Burns SB. *American Surgery: An Illustrated History* (Lippincott, Williams and Wilkins: Baltimore, 1998).

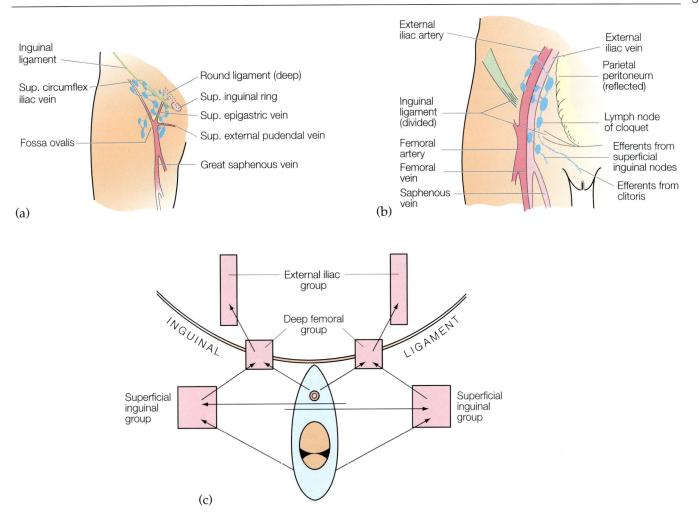

Figure 1.6 Depiction of inguinal nodes (a) and pelvic nodes (b) by Stanley Way[8] in 1951. The relationship of the nodal groups, including direct clitoral drainage to 'deep femoral' nodes and contralateral labial drainage, shown by Way in schematic form (c).

Although Way was incorrect in his assessment, he did make a prophetic plea for the establishment of special treatment centers for patients with vulvar cancer because of its rarity, the difficulty of radical surgery for vulvar cancer, and the need for experienced medical and nursing care. Way foreshadowed both the formation of the subspecialty of gynecologic oncology and the establishment of comprehensive cancer centers.

IN VIVO INJECTION OF DYES

The next advances in the study of lymphatic anatomy and the development of lymphatic mapping came from in vivo studies. Intraoperative observation of the lymphatics has always been hampered by two facts: the lymphatics are essentially invisible, and the lymph is colorless. Two of the first investigators to use living subjects for study were Stephen Hudack and Phillip McMaster.[9] They experimented with injecting a variety of vital dyes into the skin of a variety of mice rats and rabbits. They then used themselves and six other volunteers as experimental subjects to study the cutaneous lymphatics of the skin and lymphatic drainage patterns. Using very fine needles, small quantities of vital blue dyes, and photographic magnification, they were able to demonstrate the fine lymphatic capillaries of the skin. They varied the type of dye and the volume injected and measured the rate of lymph transport (up to 15 cm in 5 min) and the impact of inflamed skin, heat, and wheal formation on lymph transport. In their examination of the effect of wheal formation, they studied one individual who responded to 'a firm stroke with a blunt instrument' with formation of a wheal within 2–3 min. The lymphatics in the region of the wheal became less effective at draining the dye.

Clinicians began to experiment with injection of a variety of dyes to help visualize lymph nodes. Gray[10] injected sky-blue dye into freshly resected skin to study cutaneous lymphatics. Zeit and Wilcoxon[11] injected India ink into the cervices of patients before surgery to assist in the visualization of pelvic lymph nodes. The authors observed that this technique aided in teaching a relatively new procedure, radical hysterectomy and pelvic lymphadenectomy. Injections of 0.5 ml of India ink into the cervix at 3 and 9 o'clock at least 8 h prior to surgery stained all of the pelvic nodes black. Braithwaite[12] injected indigo

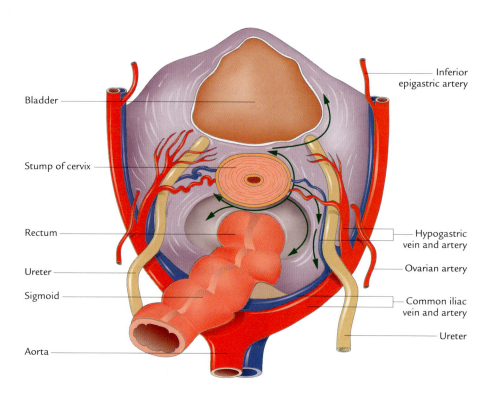

Figure 1.7 Lymphatic drainage of the cervix as depicted by Eduard Eichner[17] in 1954.

carmine into the cecum in an attempt to link appendicitis and duodenal ulcers. Weinberg and Greaney[13] injected sky blue into the peritoneum during radical gastrectomy to assist the pathologists in identification of draining lymph nodes in the specimen.

Eduard Eichner systematically studied the anatomy of the female lower genital tract using intraoperative injections of blue dyes. In a remarkable 2-year period, he published three papers that described anatomic findings after injections in the cervix, ovary, uterine fundus, vulva, and vagina[14-16] (Figure 1.7). He supplemented his work with a fourth study published in 1958, of patients with cervical stumps.[17] Eichner experimented with obstructing lymphatic flow at various points—for example, he tied off the infundibulopelvic ligament to see how this would alter lymphatic flow. Eichner made several important observations; however, he also made errors that contributed to misconceptions about lymphatic drainage of the genital tract, in particular the vulva. Eichner engaged in a series of injections of various vulvar sites. Unlike Hudack and McMaster, who used intradermal injections, Eichner used deep subcutaneous injections. Eichner was unable to demonstrate dye in the inguinal nodes of his subjects; rather, he found dye in the pelvic nodes. Presumably, the dye was following the prevascular lymphatics of the deep vessels of the vulva directly to the pelvis rather than following the superficial cutaneous lymphatics that drain the groin. This work suggested direct lymphatic drainage from the vulva to the pelvis. It took several decades to demonstrate that this very rarely, if ever, occurs.

EARLY EFFORTS AT SENTINEL NODE IDENTIFICATION

The individual most frequently credited with coining the phrase 'sentinel node' is Ernest Gould.[1] He proposed using the lymph node found at the junction of the anterior and posterior facial veins for frozen-section analysis to determine the need for a full neck dissection. His hypothesis, based on findings in 28 patients with parotid cancer, was that if this node was negative, the remaining lymph nodes of the neck would also be negative and full neck dissection could be avoided.

The individual who combined the two elements of the modern approach, lymphatic mapping and sentinel node identification, is Ramon Cabanas. Cabanas, along with Manuel Riveros and Ramiro Garcia, first described lymphography of the penis in a 1967 report of an anatomic study performed while Cabanas was at the National University in Asunción, Paraguay.[18] Paraguay has one of the highest incidences of penile carcinoma in the world. Cabanas later did a fellowship in urologic oncology at Memorial Sloan-Kettering Cancer Center. Over an 8-year period, Cabanas amassed a series of 80 patients with penile cancer in whom he used lymphography to identify the sentinel lymph node in the groin (Figure 1.8). He found that the sentinel lymph node was always located among the superficial inguinal nodes, that the sentinel node was involved with disease in all patients who had metastases, and that the sentinel node was the only positive node in 12 cases. Cabanas suggested that only the patients with a positive sentinel lymph node required the more extensive (and morbid) procedure of complete lymphadenectomy.

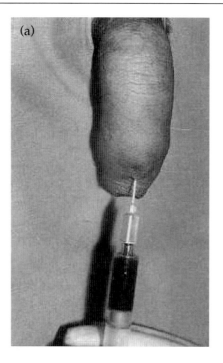

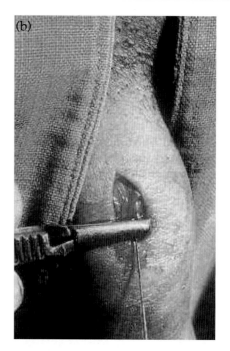

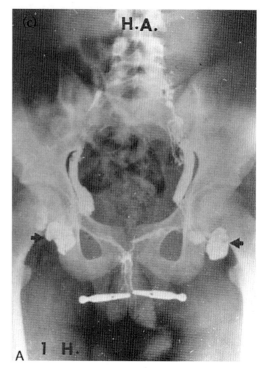

Figure 1.8 Cabanas' technique for penile lymphography. Blue dye injected into the phallus of the penis is taken up by cutaneous lymphatics. A cut-down is performed and the dorsal lymphatic is canalized and injected with ethiodized oil. Plain radiographs identify both the lymphatic channel and ethoidized oil deposited in the sentinel node. (Reproduced from *Cancer* with permission[18]).

In the 1970s, Cabanas was conducting his studies of sentinel nodes in patients with penile cancer, while gynecologic oncologists were attempting to find ways to reduce the morbidity of radical vulvectomy and bilateral inguinal femoral lymphadenectomy. Parry-Jones[19] performed in vivo injections of blue dye to show that vulvar lymphatics do not cross the buttock and labial-crural fold, as had been depicted by Sappey. This observation permitted surgeons to reduce the radicality of the operation while still adhering to Halstedian principles. In contrast to Eichner, Parry-Jones used intradermal injections and found in all cases that the dye was arrested in the groin and did not reach the pelvic nodes. This conflicted with his hypothesis that there is direct lymphatic drainage from the vulva to the pelvis. Rather than reject his hypothesis, Parry-Jones rejected his methods. After experimenting with several compounds, he settled on Imferon injected into the subcutaneous tissue of the vulva 24 h prior to surgery. Iron particles found in the iliac lymph nodes confirmed for Parry-Jones his hypothesis that the vulva has lymphatic drainage directly to the pelvic nodes.[19]

Other investigators took other avenues to reduce the morbidity of radical vulvectomy and bilateral inguinal femoral lymphadenectomy. Wharton et al[20] suggested that the risk of lymph node metastases in patients with less than 5-mm invasion was so low that lymphadenectomy could be omitted in these patients. This approach was rapidly abandoned, however, following the subsequent publication of several reports of lymph node metastases in patients with less than 5-mm invasion.[21] Morris[22] suggested that patients with well-lateralized lesions could be treated with hemivulvectomy. This work represented one of the earliest departures from the practice of performing radical vulvectomy for treatment of invasive vulvar cancer and was a clear departure from the Halstedian concept of en bloc resection.

Philip DiSaia focused the attention of the gynecologic oncology community on the devastating effect of radical vulvectomy on body image and sexual function. In 1979, he described combining less radical resection of the primary tumor with a less radical approach to groin dissection, as suggested by Cabanas. DiSaia proposed radical local excision and superficial inguinal lymphadenectomy for selected patients with vulvar cancer.[23] DiSaia introduced the term 'sentinel nodes' to the gynecologic oncology community in North America. DiSaia suggested that the superficial inguinal lymph nodes were the sentinel nodes of the vulva. This is the location where Cabanas always found the sentinel nodes in patients with penile cancer, and DiSaia added his own observation that the femoral nodes were never positive if the superficial inguinal nodes were negative. DiSaia relied on location relative to anatomic landmarks to identify 'sentinel nodes'—a technique similar to that described by Gould in 1960—rather than relying on landmarks in combination with lymphatic mapping, as described by Cabanas. The sentinel node concept proposed by DiSaia in 1978 has been investigated by several other groups with mixed results. Berman et al[24] reported no groin relapses in a group of 50 cervical cancer patients. This is in contrast to the results of Gynecologic Oncology Group (GOG) protocol 75, reported by Stehman et al,[25] in which almost 8% of the 121 patients with vulvar cancer suffered a groin recurrence following superficial inguinal lymphadenectomy with negative nodes. This compares with a recurrence rate of less than 1% following inguinal femoral lymphadenectomy with negative nodes in a group of more than 300 patients participating in GOG protocol 37.[26] On the basis of the GOG results, most gynecologic oncologists have abandoned superficial inguinal lymphadenectomy as it was described by DiSaia in 1978.

PROGRESS TOWARD THE MODERN LYMPHATIC MAPPING CONCEPT

Injection of radionuclides into human subjects to localize regional lymph nodes was first reported in 1953 by Sherman and Ter-Pogossian.[27] Numerous radiolabeled compounds have since been used for this purpose. The first gynecologic application of lymphoscintigraphy was in 1982, when Iversen and Aas[28] studied vulvar lymphatic drainage in a group of 52 patients, most of whom had cervix cancer. A group led by Donald Morton developed the first important clinical application of lymphoscintigraphy by using colloidal gold to identify the primary nodal drainage basin in patients with cutaneous melanoma at sites on the body with ambiguous lymphatic drainage patterns, primarily the trunk (Figure 1.9).

At this time of Morton's studies, there was a major debate regarding the management of patients with early-stage melanoma. The vast majority of these patients, 90%, have negative nodes, and the efficacy of regional lymphadenectomy in the 10% with positive nodes was the subject of intense debate. Some clinicians recommended a complete lymphadenec-

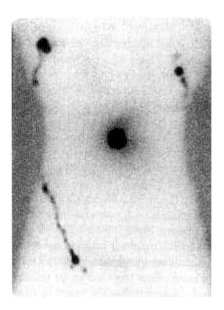

Figure 1.9 Lymphoscintogram of a patient with a cutaneous melanoma of the midback. Note lymphatic drainage to three of four potential lymphatic basins (from Nieweg O, Jansen L, Uren RF, et al, *Instructive Cases: Case 4: Drainage to Multiple Basins*. In Nieweg O, Essner R, Reintgen D, eds, *Lymphatic Mapping and Probe Applications in Oncology* (Marcel Dekker, Inc.: New York, 2000) 292–4.)

tomy in all patients with stage I disease, while others recommended observation. Morton set out to determine whether the sentinel node as described by Cabanas and others could be identified intraoperatively. His group studied various dyes in a feline model[29] and selected isosulfan blue as the best choice for intraoperative lymphatic mapping. In 1992, Morton et al[30] described their results in 223 patients with cutaneous melanoma. A total of 237 lymphatic basins were mapped, and the sentinel node was identified in 82% of them. More than 3000 lymph nodes were removed, of which 8% were sentinel, and in only two cases did nonsentinel nodes contain metastatic disease when the sentinel nodes were disease free. This paper is one of the most cited references in modern surgical oncology and prompted an explosion of interest in this technique.

In rapid succession, several large series of lymphatic mapping and sentinel node biopsy in patients with breast cancer and melanoma were published from centers around the world, essentially all confirming Morton et al's observations. A decade later, reports have been published describing lymphatic mapping and sentinel node identification in patients with head and neck, endocrine, gastrointestinal, genitourinary, and reproductive cancers. At least 40 validation trials using various techniques have been conducted in patients with breast cancer, with an overall predictive value of negative sentinel nodes of 96%.[31] In addition, several multi-institutional phase III trials are now under way in breast cancer and melanoma patients, comparing sentinel node biopsy with or without regional lymphadenectomy.

Just 2 years after Morton's first description of lymphatic mapping in patients with cutaneous melanoma, the first gynecologic application of his blue dye technique was reported.[32] Since then, a large body of literature describing lymphatic mapping and sentinel node identification has ensued. The following chapters will review this literature in detail.

REFERENCES

1. Gould EA, Winship T, Philbin PH, Hyland Kerr H. Observations on a 'sentinel node' in cancer of the parotid. *Cancer* 1960;**13**:77–8.
2. Leveuf J, Godard H. Les lymphatiques de l'utérus. *Rev Chir* 1923;219–48.
3. Borgstein P, Meijer S. Historical perspective of lymphatic tumour spread and the emergence of the sentinel node concept. *Eur J Surg Oncol* 1998;**24**:85–9.
4. Plentl AA, Friedman EA. Lymphatics of the cervix uteri. In: *Lymphatic System of Female Genitalia* (WB Saunders: Philadelphia, 1971) 75–115.
5. Twombly G. The technique of radical vulvectomy for carcinoma of the vulva. *Cancer* 1953;**3**:516–30.
6. Taussig FJ. Cancer of the vulva: an analysis of 155 cases. *Am J Obstet Gynecol* 1940;**40**:764–73.
7. Way S. Carcinoma of the vulva. *Am J Obstet Gynecol* 1960;**79**:692.

8. Way S. Carcinoma of the vulva. In: *Malignant Disease of the Female Genital Tract* (Blakiston, Philadelphia, 1951) 27–8.

9. Hudack S, McMaster P. The lymphatic participation in human cutaneous phenomena. *J Exp Med* 1933;**57**:751–74.

10. Gray J. The relation of lymphatic vessels to the spread of cancer. *Br J Surg* 1938;**6**:462–95.

11. Zeit PR, Wilcoxon G. In vivo coloring of pelvic lymph nodes with India ink. *Am J Obstet Gynecol* 1950;**59**:1164–6.

12. Braithwaite L. Flow of lymph from iliocecal angle. *Br J Surg* 1923;**11**:7.

13. Weinberg JA, Greaney EM. Identification of regional lymph nodes by means of a vital staining during surgery of gastric cancer. *Surg Gyn Obst* 1950;**90**:561–5.

14. Eichner E, Bove ER. In vivo studies on the lymphatic drainage of the human ovary. *Obstet Gynecol* 1954;**3**:287–97.

15. Eichner, E. Goldberg I, Bove ER. In vivo studies with direct sky blue of the lymphatic drainage of the internal genitals of women. *Am J Obstet Gynecol* 1954;**67**:1277–1286.

16. Eichner E, Mallin LP, Angell ML. Further experience with direct sky blue in the in vivo studies of gynecologic lymphatics. *Am J Obstet Gynecol* 1955;**69**:1019–1026.

17. Eichner E, Rubinstein L. Cervical stump lymphatics. *Obstet Gynecol* 1958;**12**:521–7.

18. Riveros M, Garcia R, Cabanas R. Lymphadenectomy of the dorsal lymphatics of the penis. *Cancer* 1967;**20**:2026–31.

19. Parry-Jones E. Lymphatics of the vulva. *J Obstet Gynaecol Br Commonwealth* 1963;**70**:751–65.

20. Wharton J, Fletcher G, Delclos L. Invasive tumors of the vagina: clinical features and management. In: Coppleson M, ed, Gynecologic Oncology: Fundamental Principles and Clinical Practice (Churchill-Livingstone: New York, 1981) 345–59.

21. Parker RT, Duncan I, Rampone J, et al. Operative management of early invasive epidermoid carcinoma of the vulva. *Am J Obstet Gynecol* 1975;**123**:349–55.

22. Morris JM. A formula for selective lymphadenectomy: its application to cancer of the vulva. *Obstet Gynecol* 1977;**50**:152–8.

23. DiSaia PJ, Creasman WT, Rich WM. An alternate approach to early cancer of the vulva. *Am J Obstet & Gynecol* 1979;**133**:825–32.

24. Berman ML, Keys H, Creasman W, et al. Survival and patterns of recurrence in cervical cancer metastatic to periaortic lymph nodes (a Gynecologic Oncology Group study). *Gynecol Oncol* 1984;**19**:8–16.

25. Stehman FB, Bundy BN, Dvoretsky PM, et al. Early stage I carcinoma of the vulva treated with ipsilateral superficial inguinal lymphadenectomy and modified radical hemivulvectomy: a prospective study of the Gynecologic Oncology Group. *Obstet Gynecol* 1992;**79**:490–7.

26. Homesley HD, Bundy BN, Sedlis A, et al. Radiation therapy versus pelvic node resection for carcinoma of the vulva with positive groin nodes. *Obstet Gynecol* 1986;**68**:733–40.

27. Sherman A, Ter-Pogossian M. Lymph-node concentration of radioactive colloidal gold following interstitial injection. *Cancer* 1953;**6**:1238–40.

28. Iversen T, Aas M. Lymph drainage from the vulva. *Gynecol Oncol* 1983;**16**:179–89.

29. Wong JH, Cagle LA, Morton DL. Lymphatic drainage of skin in a sentinel lymph node in a feline model. *Ann Surg* 1991;**214**:637–41.

30. Morton DL, Wen DR, Wong JH, et al. Technical details of intraoperative lymphatic mapping for early stage melanoma. *Arch Surg* 1992;**127**:392–9.

31. Liberman L, Cody HS III, Hill ADK, et al. Sentinel lymph node biopsy after percutaneous diagnosis of nonpalpable breast cancer. *Radiology* 1999;**211**:835–44.

32. Levenback C, Morris M, Burke TW, et al. Groin dissection practices among gynecologic oncologists treating early vulvar cancer. *Gynecol Oncol* 1996;**62**:73–7.

2 LYMPHATIC ANATOMY

2a   Microanatomy and physiology of the human lymphatic system   17

2b   Lymphatic anatomy of the vulva for sentinel node mapping   27

2c   Lymphatic anatomy of the cervix   41

2d   Lymphatics of the corpus uteri   49

2e   Lymphatics of the ovary   55

2f   Lymphatic anatomy of the breast and axilla   59

2a MICROANATOMY AND PHYSIOLOGY OF THE HUMAN LYMPHATIC SYSTEM

CHARLES LEVENBACK

EARLY STUDIES OF THE LYMPHATIC SYSTEM

Introduction

The human lymphatic system is a complicated, multifunction network of lymphatic channels and lymph nodes. This system helps maintain interstitial and intravascular equilibrium, helps clear the body of various types of particulate matter, and plays a crucial immunologic role in the body's response to infection and cancer. The purpose of this chapter is to provide an overview of the lymphatic system with emphasis on how it relates to lymphatic mapping.

Up to the late nineteenth century, the study of the lymphatic system was limited to cadavers. Sappey and others used petrified tissue for dissection of lymphatic systems, but this was not suitable for histologic analysis. In the 1890s, the great physiologist E.H. Starling made important observations about the in vivo activity of lymph fluid and lymphatics. He described the interactive effects of hydrostatic and oncotic pressure on lymph flow. He also showed that lymph fluid ultimately returned to the bloodstream.[1]

The clinical use of surgery grew at the start of the twentieth century, and intraoperative observations stimulated interest in lymphatic function. Braithwaite[2] observed that pigmented lymph nodes from an infected appendix could be followed along the superior mesenteric artery to the duodenum. He speculated that appendicitis could account for duodenal and gastric ulcers.

In 1938, Gray pointed out the limits of studying decomposed tissue and began to study freshly resected skin, using injections of small amounts of a colloidal material, thorium oxide (Thorotrast).[3] This permitted a detailed study of the histology of the lymphatics of the skin. Gray defined histologic criteria for identifying lymphatics, including 1) endothelial lining, 2) frequent semilunar valves, 3) connection of lymph vessels to lymph glands, and 4) the presence of coagulated lymph or nothing in the lymph channels.[3]

Gray next injected thorium oxide into freshly resected tumors, primarily of the breast. His studies led to the conclusion that 'the mode of spread of cancer to lymph glands is generally by means of lymphatic emboli of cancer cells carried along the lymph stream'.[3] The concept that solid tumors metastasize to lymph nodes via lymphatics in an orderly manner has been the basis of the treatment of solid tumors for most of the twentieth century. This concept has been challenged by Fisher and Fisher[4] and others, who suggest that, for example, breast cancer is a systemic, not a regional, disease from the time of onset. More recently, it has been suggested that hematogenous spread is common in breast cancer; however, in most patients, regional lymph node involvement precedes systemic disease, and in some patients local-regional therapy is effective[5,6] (Table 2a.1).

LYMPH AND LYMPHATIC VESSELS

Lymphatic vessels are found in every organ of the body except bone marrow, the central nervous system, liver lobules, and spleen.[7] The lymphatic system begins with small lymphatic capillaries (terminal lymphatics) that have blind ends. These blind ends are lined by a single layer of overlapping endothelial cells with fenestration that range in size from 10 to 25 μm[8] (Figure 2a.1). These cells are anchored by collagen filaments to the surrounding connective tissue. Fluid and particles enter the lymphatic capillaries because of hydrostatic and colloidal pressure gradients or diapedesis. In response to local conditions, the anchoring collagen filaments contract or relax to open or close the spaces between the endothelial cells. In this way, these gaps act as microvalves between the lymphatic system and the interstitium. The interendothelial cell junctions are relatively large, making the terminal lymphatics highly permeable to large proteins and particulate matter. Rising luminal pressure causes the overlapping spaces to close, preventing leakage into the interstitial spaces.

Table 2a.1 Models for spread of breast cancer. (Modified with permission from *Surgical Clinics of North America*.[10])

Halsted
- Tumors spread in orderly pattern to lymph nodes
- Lymph node metastases can result in distant spread
- Lymph nodes are barriers to passage of tumor cells
- Hematogenous spread minor significance
- Extent of surgery and technique determine outcome
- Operable breast cancer is a local-regional disease

Systemic[4]
- No orderly pattern to metastases
- Lymph nodes ineffective barrier to spread
- Hematogenous spread very important
- Local regional therapy has small impact on survival
- Operable breast cancer is systemic disease

Spectrum[5]
- Axillary node spread usually precedes distant spread
- Lymph nodes ineffective barrier to spread
- Lymph node metastases not always associated with distant spread
- Hematogenous spread route for distant metastases
- Early local treatment vital to prevent distant spread
- Operable breast cancer is systemic in small proportion of patients

The terminal lymphatic capillaries drain to afferent (collecting) lymphatic channels. These afferent lymphatic channels are also semipermeable; however, they have valves every 2–3 mm and have some elastic fibers in the wall of the vessels that are two or three cells thick. These vessels join even larger vessels that ultimately drain to regional lymph nodes. The distance between valves becomes larger as the lymphatic channel becomes larger. Valves may be located every 2–3 mm in smaller lymphatics and every 6–12 mm in larger ducts.[9] The larger afferent channels have a circular layer of smooth muscle cells (Figure 2a.2).

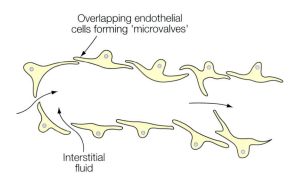

Figure 2a.1   Blind terminal sacs of lymphatic capillaries with single overlapping layer of endothelial cells. These are 10–25 μm in diameter and allow interstitial fluid to pass in and out of the lymphatic capillary. (Modified from Kam and Uren[9]).

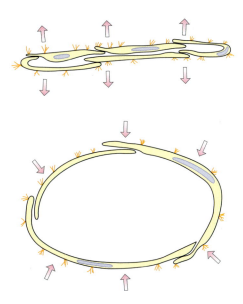

Figure 2a.2   Terminal lymphatics drain to afferent (collecting) lymphatics that are characterized by thicker walls with some contractile capability and valves, resulting in unidirectional flow. (Schmid-Schonbein GW, Microlymphatics and lymph flow, *Physiol Rev* (1990) **70**:987–1020.)

PHYSIOLOGY

Management of interstitial fluid depends on several factors, including hydrostatic pressure, osmotic pressure, diffusion and convection, and chemotaxis.[10] In response to pressure and volume conditions, the anchoring filaments of the terminal lymphatics pull apart the endothelial cells, allowing entry of interstitial fluid and debris. A variety of factors propel lymph fluid through the channels. These factors differ from place to place and include external compression by skeletal muscle, respiration, intestinal peristalsis, and intrinsic contractile mechanisms. Neurohormonal transmitters may also play a role.

The body makes 2–4 liters of lymphatic fluid a day. Under normal conditions, lymph is colorless, and the flow in lymphatic channels is unidirectional. The arterial system relies on the heart to pump fluid in a pulsatile manner; however, the lymphatics, like the veins, rely on a series of valves, external compression, and very limited intrinsic contractility to propel lymph against gravity and back towards the heart. Lymphatic vessels have very low pressure and are sensitive to small changes. It takes only 2–4 cm of H_2O to initiate rhythmic contractions of the lymphatic vessels.[11] Gray massaged tissue after injection to accelerate lymphatic flow. Many clinicians still perform external massage during lymphatic mapping to enhance dispersal of dye.

The volume, rate of flow, and composition of lymph vary with site and activity. For example, the concentration of lipids in the intestinal lymph fluid increases after a meal. In general, it can be stated that the majority of cells in lymphatic fluid are small lymphocytes, and the majority of the proteins in lymphatic fluid are plasma proteins.

A major clinical concern for those interested in lymphatic mapping is how fast lymph moves within the lymphatic system. Most recently, this was studied by Uren and colleagues in patients with cutaneous melanoma undergoing lymphoscintigraphy.[12] Peritumoral injections were made with antimony sulfide colloid labeled with technetium-99m (^{99m}Tc), and then the tumor area was immediately scanned. The flow rates varied by anatomic location, with the lowest rate observed in the head and neck and the highest observed in the lower extremity. The authors found that faster lymphatic drainage was strongly associated with uptake to second-tier (or second-echelon) nodes. Antimony sulfide has a small particle size of 10–15 nm in diameter. Sulfur microcolloid, commonly used in North America, has a larger particle size and therefore somewhat slower uptake.

From a gynecologic perspective, the primary tumor in patients with vulvar and cervix cancer is relatively close to the regional lymph node bed, and therefore radionuclide should be transferred relatively quickly to the sentinel node or nodes. An exception may be perineal primary tumors, which could be up to 10 cm from the sentinel node or nodes. Blue dyes are taken up and transferred quickly to sentinel lymph nodes. Inflammatory processes in the skin may accelerate uptake because of increase blood and lymphatic flow.

LYMPH NODES

Spread throughout the body are small, bean-shaped lymph nodes (Figure 2a.3). The lymph nodes act as a filter for particulate matter, antigens, and cancer cells. But lymph nodes are not simply filters; they are also the primary antigen recognition site in the body.[10]

The lymph fluid enters the node through the afferent lymphatic channel, described earlier. The fluid first enters into the medullary sinus. Small metastases are commonly found in this area. The lymph fluid flows through the medulla and germinal centers of the lymph node before exiting out the efferent channel, which exits the node and is formed by the merger of the medullary sinuses. This efferent channel most likely becomes the afferent channel of another lymph node in the chain or basin. All the lymphatics of the lower extremities and pelvis ultimately form large collecting ducts and ultimately form the thoracic duct. The thoracic duct passes through the chest and ultimately joins the venous system at the junction of the left subclavian vein and jugular (Figure 2a.4). This presumably accounts for the left supraclavicular lymph nodes being a common site for metastases from gynecologic cancers.

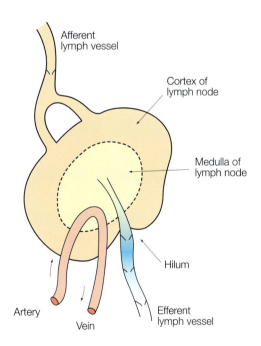

Figure 2a.3 Anatomy of a lymph node. Lymph nodes filter debris from lymph and are a critical site of antigen presentation and immune activation. (Modified from Kam and Uren[9]).

If lymph nodes recognize an antigen, a variety of events are set in motion, including activation of B and T cells for production of antibodies and cytotoxins. The lymph nodes may enlarge (this is a common clinical finding in patients with localized infections of soft-tissue structures).

The relationship between lymph node metastasis rates and primary tumor size varies from site to site. It is common to find metastases larger than the primary tumor in patients with carcinoid. Sarcomas have a low rate of regional nodal spread and a high rate of hematogenous spread. Colon cancer can spread to the liver with or without nodal spread. Lymph node status is the single most important prognostic factor in patients with squamous carcinoma of the vulva and cervix, and in patients with endometrial adenocarcinoma. Nonlymphatic modes of spread are much less common in patients with these tumors.

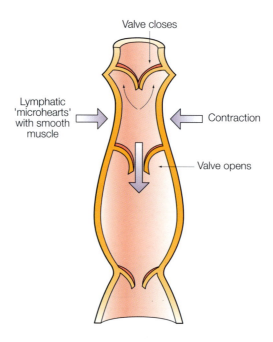

Figure 2a.4 Main lymphatic collecting trunks have valves that ensure unidirectional flow. (Modified from Kam and Uren[9]).

IMMUNOLOGY OF REGIONAL LYMPH NODES

Prior to development of lymphatic mapping, investigators sought to identify differential immunologic response within lymph nodes based on their distance from the primary tumor. Hoon et al[13] found that lymph nodes closer to the primary tumor (melanoma or breast) were less responsive to immunostimulation than those lymph nodes further away. This suggested that tumor-derived products were immunosuppressing the adjacent draining lymph nodes. In 1989, the same group described that 14% of patients with stage I melanoma had occult tumor cells in the lymph nodes on a 'direct lymphatic pathway' not detected by routine HE staining.[14] Additional studies suggested that melanoma-derived materials downregulated the immune response of these lymph nodes, increasing their susceptibility to metastasis. In another study, Farzad et al[15] took lymph node lymphocytes (LNL) and tested these LNLs against melanoma cell lines to determine their ability to inhibit tumor growth. LNLs taken from close to primary tumors inhibited growth in vivo less than lymphocytes from more distant lymph nodes.

In 2000, Almand and colleagues[16] showed that dendritic cell function was defective in cancer patients, and that this might be a factor in the metastatic process. Essner and Kojima[17] have been looking at dendritic cell function in sentinel and nonsentinel lymph nodes of melanoma patients. They found a marked reduction in the number of dendritic cells and dendritic cell activation markers in sentinel nodes compared with the paired nonsentinel node. These studies suggest that sentinel nodes are the site of first metastasis on immunologic, as well as physiologic and anatomic, grounds.

Alessandro Santin[18] recently provided an outstanding discussion of the role of regional lymphadenectomy in light of recent observations regarding cytotoxic T-cell (CTL) activation experiments. This work suggests that cytotoxic T cells are activated by the recognition of tumor antigens only after tumor cells are at least partially degraded in regional draining lymph nodes. 'It is only during the interaction between T cells and tumor cells in an environment that enhances antitumor response (i.e., the lymph nodes) that antigenic tumors become immunogenic enough to induce recognition and activation of the antigen specific, naïve T cells'.[18] Although this activation is rarely complete, this analysis raises questions about a treatment plan that includes removal of immunocompetent lymph nodes along with lymph nodes with metastatic disease and tumor-induced immune suppression.

There has been very little work along these lines in patients with gynecologic cancers. Investigators have found that human papilloma virus (HPV)-activated dendritic cells can lead to cytotoxic T-cell killing of autologous tumor cells.[19,20] Van Trappen et al[21] identified cytokeratin 19 in the regional lymph nodes of radical hysterectomy patients. Much more work is required in these areas to understand fully the metastatic process in sentinel lymph nodes and how to use this knowledge in treatment strategies.

SURGICAL ANATOMY OF THE LYMPHATIC SYSTEM

Lymphatic channels are usually not visible during surgery and are frequently disrupted without any adverse consequence to the patient. There is a large network of low-pressure lymphatic vessels and extensive collateral flow. It is uncommon to see lymphatic fluid during surgery, as the fluid is colorless and leaks slowly into the field, mixing with blood and other fluids. Lymph nodes vary in size and consistency so that some, but not all, nodes are visible or palpable during surgery.

From a surgeon's point of view, it is interesting that the number of regional lymph nodes described in surgical pathology reports varies wildly for a given procedure. Node counts are important because they are frequently interpreted as an indication of the adequacy of surgery by surgeons as well as by radiation and medical oncologists. Low node counts have caused more than one surgeon to lament, 'But I did the same procedure I always do!' In addition to surgical skill, factors that influence the node count include anatomic variation from patient to patient and the skill and persistence of the pathologist in finding the lymph nodes within the fatty tissue. Some pathologists do not report the number of lymph nodes on the grounds that counts are unreliable.

Patients with more extensive lymph node dissections are at risk of wound complications, including infection and lymphocyst. Most lymphocysts can be managed with closed-suction drainage; however, some will recur and require more aggressive intervention. This usually means surgical drainage. Large lymphocysts in the pelvis can be 'unroofed' and drained internally. An alternative is some sort of sclerosis; however, this procedure meets with mixed results.

Lymphedema is the most troubling complication of lymphadenectomy. Lymphedema occurs when there is extensive disruption of lymphatic drainage that leads to an increase in the lymphatic pressure required to bypass the obstructed site, resulting in accumulation of lymph in the tissue. In gynecologic patients, lymphedema is most often seen in the lower extremities (Figure 2a.5). Factors that can contribute to lymphedema following regional lymphadenectomy include more extensive surgery and delivery of postoperative radiation therapy. Unfortunately, options for treatment of lymphedema are limited. Compression hose, sequential compression devices, massage, and simple elevation all can help control lymphedema but cannot fully reverse it.

SUMMARY

Understanding of the physiologic molecular and immunologic events taking place within lymph nodes continues to expand. Lymphatic mapping and sentinel node biopsy provide an opportunity to narrow the focus of basic science and translational, as well as clinical, investigation. We hope that innovations in treating gynecologic cancers will follow advances in knowledge of sentinel and nonsentinel lymph nodes.

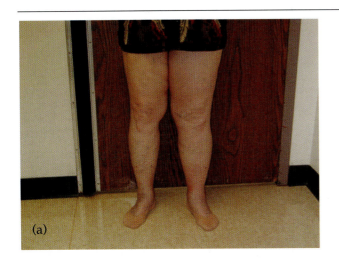

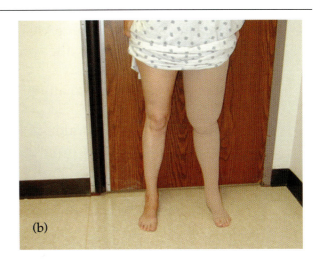

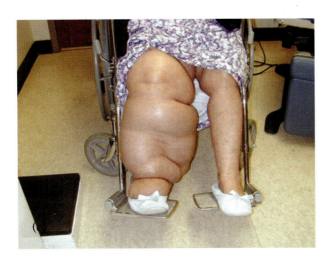

Figure 2a.5 Various degrees of lymphedema. Mild lymphedema (a) causes little effect on lifestyle. Moderate lymphedema (b) requires compression devices and massage; however, most patients continue to function well. Severe lymphedema (c) is debilitating.

REFERENCES

1. Starling E. On the absorption of fluid from the connective tissue spaces. *J Physiol (Lond)* 1896;**19**:312–26.
2. Braithwaite L. Flow of lymph from iliocecal angle. *Br J Surg* 1923;**11**:7.
3. Gray J. The relation of lymphatic vessels to the spread of cancer. *Br J Surg* 1938;**26**:462–95.
4. Fisher B, Fisher ER. The interrelationship of hematogenous and lymphatic tumor cell dissemination. *Surg Gynecol Obstet* 1966;**122**:791–8.
5. Harris J, Hellman S. Natural history of breast cancer. In: Harris Jr LM, Morrow M, et al, eds, *Diseases of the Breast* (Lippincott-Raven: Philadelphia 1996) 375–91.

6. Koscielny S, Tubiana M, Le MG, et al. Breast cancer: relationship between the size of the primary tumour and the probability of metastatic dissemination. *Br J Cancer* 1984;**49**:709–15.

7. Foster RS Jr. General anatomy of the lymphatic system. *Surg Oncol Clin North Am* 1996;**5**:1–13.

8. Tanis PJ, Nieweg OE, Valdes Ólmos RA, et al. Anatomy and physiology of lymphatic drainage of the breast from the perspective of sentinel node biopsy. *J Am Coll Surg* 2001;**192**:399–409.

9. Kam C, Uren RF. Microanatomy and physiology of the lymphatic system. In: Nieweg O, et al, eds, *Lymphatic Mapping and Probe Applications in Oncology* (Marcel Dekker: New York, 2000) 1–22.

10. Gervasoni JE Jr, Taneja C, Chung MA, et al. Biologic and clinical significance of lymphadenectomy. *Surg Clin North Am* 2000;**80**:1631–73.

11. Aukland K, Reed RK. Interstitial-lymphatic mechanisms in the control of extracellular fluid volume. *Physiol Rev* 1993;**73**:1–78.

12. Uren RF, Howman-Giles RB, Thompson JF. Demonstration of second-tier lymph nodes during preoperative lymphoscintigraphy for melanoma: incidence varies with primary tumor site. *Ann Surg Oncol* 1998;**5**:517–21.

13. Hoon DS, Korn EL, Cochran AJ. Variations in functional immunocompetence of individual tumor-draining lymph nodes in humans. *Cancer Res* 1987;**47**:1740–4.

14. Cochran AJ, Wen DR, Farzad Z, et al. Immunosuppression by melanoma cells as a factor in the generation of metastatic disease. *Anticancer Res* 1989;**9**:859–64.

15. Farzad Z, McBride WH, Ogbechi H, et al. Lymphocytes from lymph nodes at different distances from human melanoma vary in their capacity to inhibit/enhance tumor cell growth in vitro. *Melanoma Res* 1997;**7**(Suppl 2):S59–65.

16. Almand B, Resser JR, Lindman B, et al. Clinical significance of defective dendritic cell differentiation in cancer. *Clin Cancer Res* 2000;**6**:1755–66.

17. Essner R, Kojima M. Dendritic cell function in sentinel nodes. *Oncology* 2002;**16** (Suppl 1):27–31.

18. Santin AD. Lymph node metastases: the importance of the microenvironment. *Cancer* 2000;**88**:175–9.

19. Santin AD, Hermonat PL, Ravaggi A, et al. Induction of human papillomavirus-specific CD4(+) and CD8(+) lymphocytes by E7-pulsed autologous dendritic cells in patients with human papillomavirus type 16- and 18-positive cervical cancer. *J Virol* 1999;**73**:5402–10.

20. Santin AD, Hermonat PL, Ravaggi A, et al. Development, characterization and distribution of adoptively transferred peripheral blood lymphocytes primed by human papillomavirus 18 E7-pulsed autologous dendritic cells in a patient with metastatic adenocarcinoma of the uterine cervix. *Eur J Gynaecol Oncol* 2000;**21**:17–23.

21. Van Trappen P, Gyselman VG, Lowe DG, et al. Molecular quantification and mapping of lymph-node micrometastases in cervical cancer. *Lancet* 2001;**357**(9249):15–20.

2b LYMPHATICS OF THE VULVA

ROBERT L. COLEMAN

THE VULVA

In certain respects, understanding the anatomy of the vulva, its targeted nodal basin, and its directed, physiologic lymphatic drainage should provide the clearest insight into why lymphatic mapping as a surgical procedure garners clinical relevance. Detailed study of this anatomy coupled with clinical correlates of patients with vulvar carcinoma has dictated surgical care, of which nodal resection in toto has become a standard procedure. This section will highlight the anatomy of the vulva and the groin, drawing on embryologic and postmortem studies, which recently have challenged the traditional concepts of nodal location and thus are important to surgical concepts guiding management.

Embryology of the vulva and the groin

Embryologically, the external female genitalia arise from undifferentiated tissues that comprise the genital tubercle, labioscrotal swellings, and urogenital folds.[1] In the absence of fetal androgens, further differentiation of these tissues forms the external female phenotype, which is distinguishable 12 weeks after fertilization. Ambiguity of this differentiation can result from the presence of exogenous or endogenous sex steroids during development; however, the null phenotype is female.

Topography of the vulva

The vulva comprises the mons pubis, the clitoris, the labia majora and minora, the vestibule (urethral meatus and hymenal remnant), the perineal body, the associated erectile tissues and muscles, and the supporting subcutaneous tissues (Figure 2b.1). Superficially, these structures consist of, or are covered by, a keratinized, stratified, squamous epithelium to the level of the vestibule, where the epidermis becomes a nonkeratinized squamous mucous membrane. The vulvar structures are situated atop the superficial perineal fascia, a caudal continuation of the abdominal Scarpa's layer. Support is given to the vulva through loose attachment to this fascia. Deep to this layer are the erectile and muscular contents of the genital floor (Figure 2b.2). The deep or inferior fascia of the urogenital diaphragm, on which the clitoris and ischiocavernosus, bulbocavernosus, and deep transverse perineal muscles lie, is an important surgical landmark indicating the deep margin of locoregional resection. This fascial layer becomes continuous with the fascia lata laterally.

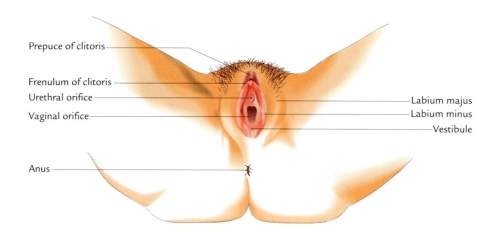

Figure 2b.1   The external female genitalia are highlighted with the major anatomic landmarks.

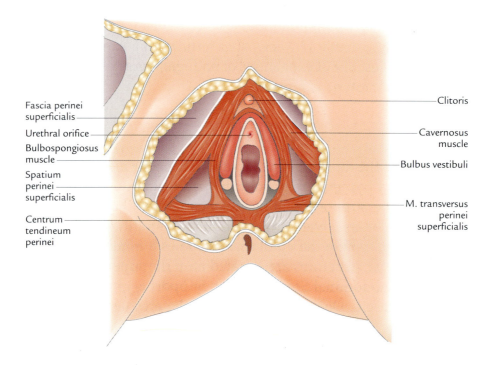

Figure 2b.2   The deep vulvar tissues are positioned in relation to the deep perineal fascia (urogenital diaphragm).

Topography of the inguinal lymphatics

The landmarks and topographic anatomy of the groin are illustrated in Figures 2b.3a, b. The same keratinizing squamous epithelium that covers the vulva, covers the groin. Deep to the skin is the subcutaneous tissue, which is divided by the superficial, or Camper's, fascia. Dorsal to this layer is fatty tissue containing the superficial inguinal nodes and the

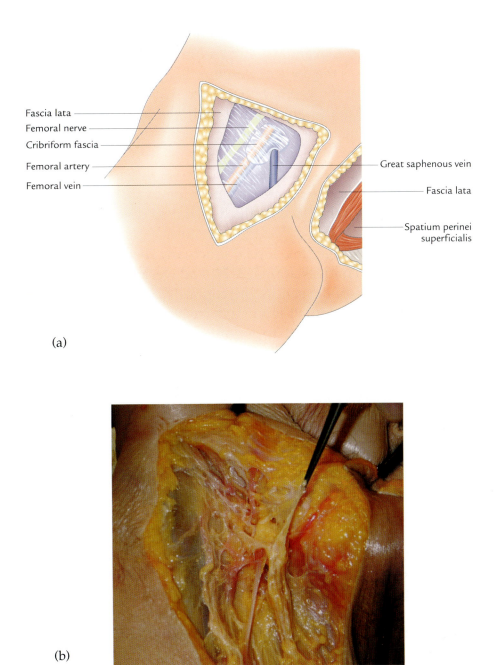

Fascia lata
Femoral nerve
Cribriform fascia
Femoral artery
Femoral vein

Great saphenous vein

Fascia lata

Spatium perinei superficialis

(a)

(b)

Figure 2b.3 The topographic anatomy of the groin is presented (right side).

superficial vasculature, such as the superficial external circumflex vessels, the superficial inferior epigastrics vessels, and the superficial external pudendal vessels. Removal of this layer reveals the deep femoral fascia, which is continuous laterally with the fascia lata of the thigh, and medially with the fascia of the adductor longus muscle, and which is coplanar with the inferior fascia of the urogenital diaphragm. The fossa ovalis is demarcated by the falciform, or Hey's, ligament and is perforated by the great saphenous vein and other small vessels. As described below, the perforate covering over the fossa is most aptly termed the cribiform lamina. Below the femoral fascia lies the femoral vessels and nerve along with the deep musculature of the groin. The femoral or deep inguinal nodes are located along the femoral vein and usually within the fossa ovalis. The most superior node is commonly referred to as the node of Rosenmüller or Cloquet. Lymphatic drainage of the vulva (and lower third of the vagina) goes principally to the groin by traversing the subcutaneous tissue medial to the labial-crural fold. The node groups are situated in the subcutaneous tissue overlying the femoral triangle (Scarpa's triangle) bounded by the inguinal ligament cephalad, the sartorius muscle inferior-laterally, and the adductor longus medially. Anatomically, these nodes are categorized as 'superficial' and 'deep' according to their location in reference to the fascia lata and position in the fossa ovalis (Figures 2b.4a, b). Traditional illustrations of the fossa ovalis depict it as covered by a perforated membrane contiguous with the fascia lata called the cribriform fascia. However, recent embryologic studies have documented that this 'fascia' is actually distinct from the fascia lata (femoral portion) and develops in midgestation (23–24 fetal weeks) from the connective tissue of the fossa ovalis.[2–4] Through condensation, the connective tissue's superficial layer becomes a thickened membrane; therefore, it is more correctly termed cribriform 'lamina.' This distinction is important and relevant to the anticipated location of the inguinal nodes, as embryologic nodal buds, which make up the deep femoral chain, arise from superficial nodes in this same connective tissue.

Superficial inguinal lymphatics

The superficial inguinal nodal group primarily receives afferent channels from the vulvar tissues traversing the labia and mons veneris. This group contains approximately 10 nodes, which lie in the subcutaneous tissue in or around the fossa ovalis and the saphenous vein and its tributaries. Detailed topographic studies of this nodal group have demonstrated that these nodes lie uniformly within Scarpa's triangle. Nicklin et al detailed this nodal group location in reference to anatomic-surgical landmarks, such as the anterior superior iliac spine and the pubic tubercle, using lymphangiography.[5] They noted that the most lateral node in this group was never positioned in the outer 15% of the right inguinal ligament or the outer 20% of the left inguinal ligament. A subsequent study by Micheletti et al correlated this observation anatomically and embryologically, as being associated with the superficial external circumflex vasculature.[3,6] In their study of preterm fetuses, nodal tissue was identified around these vessels and never lateral to the crossing of the medial border of the sartorius muscle and the inguinal ligament. The surgical implications of these

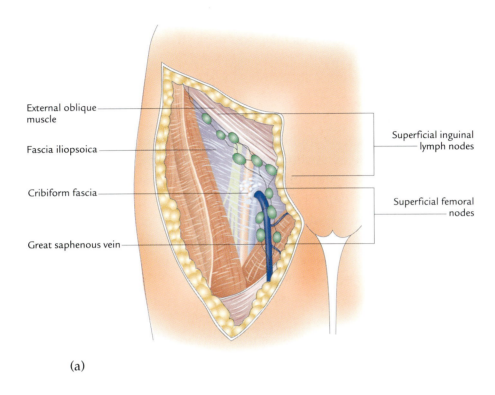

External oblique
muscle

Fascia iliopsoica

Cribiform fascia

Great saphenous vein

Superficial inguinal
lymph nodes

Superficial femoral
nodes

(a)

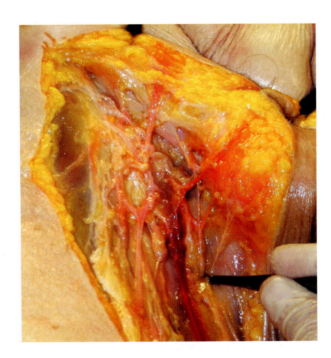

(b)

Figure 2b.4 The superficial inguinal nodes are illustrated in relationship to the femoral fascia and fossa ovalis.

findings support limiting the lateral extent of the skin and groin nodal dissection, which in turn may reduce operative morbidity by not disrupting important potential collateral lymphatic flow. Medially and inferiorly, the superficial bundle is limited by the femoral triangle.

Femoral (deep) inguinal lymphatics

The femoral or deep nodes, as mentioned, develop embryologically from a nodal mass, which is situated by 11 weeks' gestation on top of the femoral fascia. During gestation, the connective tissue of the fossa proliferates and differentiates, dividing the nodal bundle into individual nodes. A few, usually 1–5 in total, migrate in the fossa to lie along the femoral vein and become the femoral nodes.[6] Cadaveric studies of the groin have found that these nodes are most often found at or below the junction of the saphenous vein with the femoral vein (Figure 2b.5). In one-third of cases, the nodal tissue is located cephalad to this point.[2] All nodal tissue appears to be bound by the margins of the fossa ovalis. No nodal tissue is found beneath the fasica lata in any direction, and it is never located lateral to the femoral artery.

Interestingly, Cloquet's node in their series was identified in just 46% of the dissections and was unilateral in 30%, rendering it an imperfect marker of cephalad nodal extent. It is hypothesized that this node's location is also variably identified as the most distal node in the external iliac chain.

Lymphatic drainage

The clinically important features of in vivo vulvar lymphatic drainage, first described by Eichner and later by Parry-Jones, are that ipsilateral flow from the vulva does not cross the labial-crural fold laterally and that, in general, only midline structures (clitoris and perineum) have bilateral efferent drainage.[7,8] Direct communication of the clitoral lymphatics to the pelvis has been demonstrated, although this is, clinically, rarely, if ever, observed.[9] Ordered lymphatic flow from the vulva generally goes to the superficial group first, followed by drainage to the femoral nodes. From there, the efferent channels pass under the inguinal ligament in the femoral canal to communicate with the external iliac and pelvic nodal chains. Lymphatic mapping studies in women undergoing groin dissection for cancer of the vulva have confirmed the variable location of the sentinel node, although it is most commonly a medially located superficial node near the fossa ovalis.[10] Confusion regarding the existence of direct vulvar lymphatic drainage to the pelvis has been confounded by different in vivo mapping techniques. However, studies that have used intradermal injection demonstrate exclusive primary lymphatic drainage to the groin. However, studies using deep subcutaneous injections have shown direct drainage to the pelvis. Clinical experience has indicated that the best candidates for lymphatic mapping of cutaneous tumors are those with small, superficial tumors that essentially have exclusive lymphatic drainage via cutaneous lymphatics.

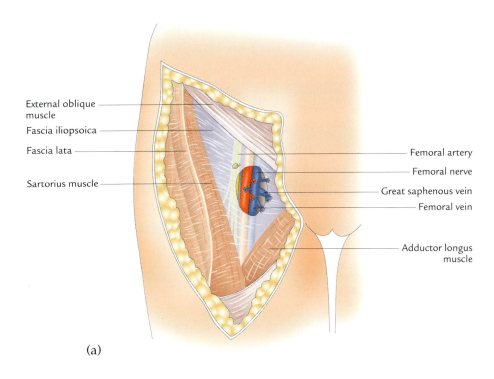

External oblique muscle

Fascia iliopsoica

Fascia lata

Sartorius muscle

Femoral artery

Femoral nerve

Great saphenous vein

Femoral vein

Adductor longus muscle

(a)

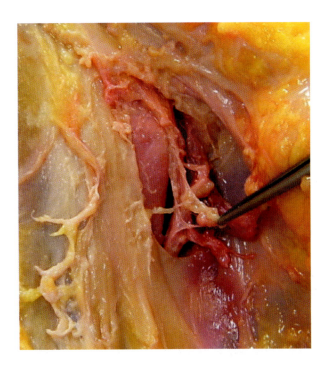

(b)

Figure 2b.5   The relationship between the deep inguinal nodes and the femoral triangle is depicted.

NATURAL HISTORY AND PATTERNS OF SPREAD

Although many tumor cell types can arise within the vulva or its associated adnexal structures, most primary carcinomas of the vulva are squamous cell and arise from the epithelium.[11] The most frequent sites of involvement are the labia minora, clitoris, fourchette, perineal body, and medial labia majora. The classic pattern of growth and spread is local extension and lymphovascular embolization to either regional or distant sites. With the exception of vulvar melanoma, the pattern of spread is relatively predictable. Local growth of the primary generally occurs in a radial pattern, as well as invading deep into the underlying subcutaneous tissues. Objective measures of this growth have been standardized with creation of the TNM staging system.[12] In this manner, tumor is described in reference to size (T1 ≤ 2 cm, T2 > 2 cm), involvement of the distal midline structures (T3: urethra, vagina and anus) and invasion of the midline organs (T4: bladder mucosa, upper urethra, and rectal mucosa), or bony fixation.

Once invasion occurs, the tumor can spread via the dermal lymphatics to the regional nodes following the previously described pattern of flow. There appears to be a threshold with regard to the likelihood of groin metastatic disease based on the depth of invasion. Kelley and colleagues reported that the frequency of metastatic disease among 24 patients with 1 mm or less of invasion (measured as depth of deepest invasion from the most proximal adjacent rete peg) was 0%.[13] This observation has led to a subclassification of stage I disease (IA: T1 lesion with 1 mm invasion or less, IB: T1 lesion with greater than 1 mm invasion), with the clinical implication being that nodal dissection may safely be dismissed in these patients.

A recent trend in the management of early vulvar cancer has been the separate resection of the primary tumor and the at-risk groin(s).[14–16] Careful inspection of en bloc tumor resections and biopsies by Cherry and Glücksmann demonstrated that tumor lymphatic emboli were present in only 19% of cases.[17] Clinically, recurrences in the retained skin bridges among patients undergoing separate incision removal of the primary lesion and the regional lymphatics are very uncommon. This observation would support the hypothesis that lymphatic metastases occur as a result of embolization rapidly and most often without interval deposition of viable tumor.

ILLUSTRATION OF THE ANATOMY OF THE GROIN

There is no other anatomic area of concern to gynecologic oncologists where so much confusion reigns regarding anatomy and nomenclature as the groin. The nomenclature issues have been explored in detail by several authors.[2,3,18] Confusion regarding nomenclature has been compounded by errors in illustration of groin anatomy that are propagated by new comment on the subject. This section we will review the efforts of previous illustrators to depict groin anatomy, as well as identify the most accurate images.

In 1971, Plentl and Friedman offered a new set of illustrations of the groin that were widely imitated[19] (Figure 2b.6a–c). In Figure 2b.6a, the general location of the superficial inguinal nodes are accurate; however, the number (5) is fewer than the 8–10 commonly found. In all the figures, the superficial and femoral nodes are shown as the same size. It is common for the nodes to vary in size; sentinel nodes are usually at least 1 cm in size. In the cross-section in Figure 2b.6c, the patient is very thin, as there is almost no fat between the

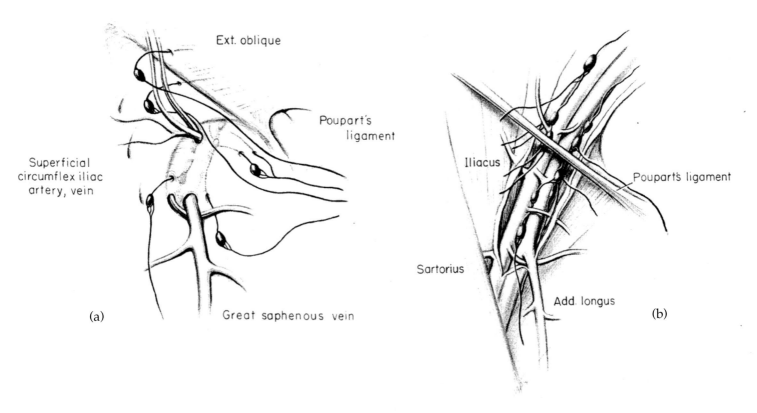

Figure 2b.6a, b, and c
Lymphatic anatomy of the right groin as demonstrated in 1971 by Plentl and Friedman,[24] (Reproduced with permission from Elsevier.)

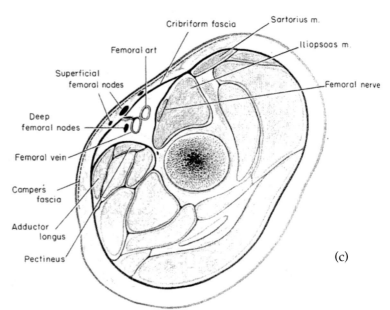

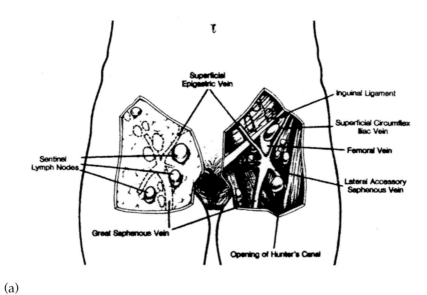

(a)

(b)

Figure 2b.7a and b Sentinel lymph nodes and inguinal femoral anatomy as illustrated by DiSaia et al,[22] (Reproduced with permission from Elsevier.)

skin and Camper's fascia. This figure shows the superficial nodes very close to the skin. In other patients, the 'superficial' inguinal nodes can be very 'deep' to the skin due to a thick layer of subcutaneous fat. This overlooked observation contributed to the poor results observed with external beam radiation therapy by the Gynecologic Oncology Group.[20] The cribriform fascia is depicted as a bold black line separating the superficial and femoral nodes. As described earlier, this structure is more appropriately described as a lamina.

Figures drawn by Cabanas[21] to illustrate the location of sentinel nodes in the male groin were modified by DiSaia et al. in 1979 to depict the location of the superficial inguinal nodes[22] (Figure 2b.7a). This figure shows the nodes as being rather large and shows 'sentinel' nodes in multiple sites. Current mapping experience suggests that sentinel nodes are usually at the medial edge of the femoral triangle and rarely lateral to the saphenous vein. DiSaia et al also introduced a new cross-section illustration of the groin (Figure 2b.7b). This illustration shows seven nodes in a single cross-section, the femoral nodes larger than the superficial nodes, the femoral nodes lateral to the femoral artery, and the cribriform fascia as a continuous thick structure. This illustration has been updated to portray more accurately cribriform fascia as fenestrated (Figure 2b.8). In addition, the traditionally described 'femoral' nodes are now within the fossa ovalis, and the distinction of these nodes as 'below' the cribriform fascia has been de-emphasized. Other texts have taken a different

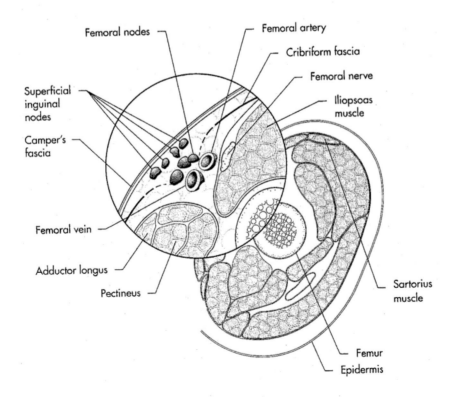

Figure 2b.8   Further update of cross-sectional anatomy of the groin.[25]

approach (Figure 2b.9a–b). In Figure 2b.9a, the lymphatics of the vulva appear to cross the labial-crural fold, contrary to the work of Parry-Jones.[7] In Figure 2b.9b, Camper's fascia is not shown, and the cribriform fascia follows an undulating path with the appearance of all the lymph nodes 'above' this structure. Recently, Rouzier et al[23] attempted to illustrate the levels of the groin schematic diagrams that show the extent of various surgical approaches (Figure 2b.10).

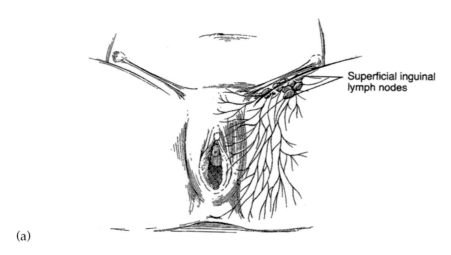

(a)

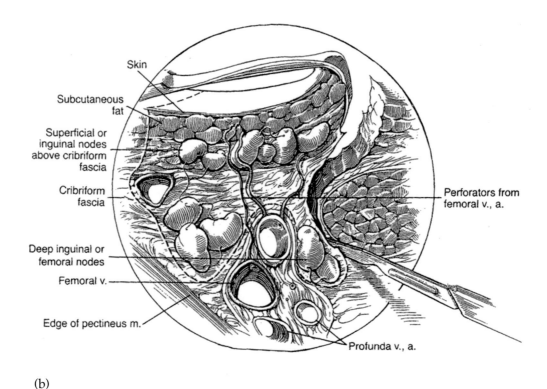

(b)

Figure 2b.9a and b Vulvar and inguinal lymphatic anatomy.[26]

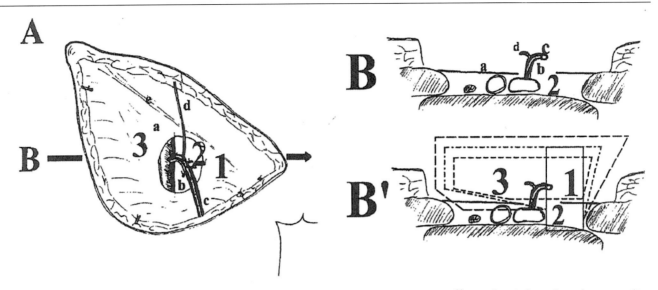

Figure 2b.10 Operative (A) and cross-sectional (B) anatomy of the groin.[23] a = fascia lata; b = fossa ovalis; c = great saphenous vein; d = superficial epigastric vein; e = inguinal ligament. The compartments of the groin are (1) superficial medial inguinal nodes, (2) medial femoral nodes, and (3) superficial lateral inguinal nodes. Sentinel nodes are most commonly found in compartment (1) and sometimes in compartment (3). Femoral sentinel nodes are rarely, if ever, seen.

SUMMARY

The anatomic considerations of the vulva and groin continue to play a vital role in the evolution of contemporary management strategies. Lymphatic mapping and sentinel node procedures have led to a better understanding of in vivo groin anatomy, particularly since the blue dye procedure allows clear visualization of lymphatic channels and lymph nodes. It is anticipated that future study will further elucidate important selection criteria whereby patients will undergo individualized curative extirpative surgery with minimal morbidity.

REFERENCES

1. Langman J. Urogenital system. In: Langman J, ed, *Medical Embryology* (William & Wilkins: Baltimore, MD, 1981) 255–9.

2. Borgno G, Micheletti L, Barbero M, et al. Topographic distribution of groin lymph nodes. *J Reprod Med* 1990;**35**:1127–9.

3. Micheletti L, Preti M, Zola P, et al. A proposed glossary of terminology related to the surgical treatment of vulvar carcinoma. *Cancer* 1998;**83**:1369–75.

4. Micheletti L, Levi AC, Bogliatto F, et al. Rationale and definition of the lateral extension of the inguinal lymphadenectomy for vulvar cancer derived from an embryological and anatomical study. *J Surg Oncol* 2002;**81**:19–24.

5. Nicklin JL, Hacker NF, Heintze SW, et al. An anatomical study of inguinal lymph nodes topography and clinical implications for the surgical management of vulval cancer. *Int J Gynecol Cancer* 1995;**5**:128–33.

6. Micheletti L, Levi AC, Bogliatto F. Anatomosurgical implications derived from an embryological study of Scarpa's triangle with particular reference to groin lymphadenectomy. *Gynecol Oncol* 1998;**70**:358–64.

7. Parry-Jones E. Lymphatics of the vulva. *J Obstet Gynecol Br Commonwealth* 1963;**70**:751–65.

8. Eichner E, Mallin LP, Angell ML. Further experience with direct sky blue in the in vivo studies of gynecic lymphatics. *Am J Obstet Gynecol* 1955;**69**:1019–26.

9. Merrill J, Ropss N. Cancer of the vulva. *Cancer* 1961;**14**:13–16.

10. Levenback C, Coleman RL, Burke TW, et al. Intraoperative lymphatic mapping and sentinel node identification with blue dye in patients with vulvar cancer. *Gynecol Oncol* 2001;**83**:276–81.

11. Wilkinson E. Premalignant and malignant tumors of the vulva. In: Kurman R, ed, *Blaustein's Pathology of the Female Genital Tract* (Springer-Verlag: New York, 1994) 87–129.

12. AJCC, *Cancer Staging Manual*. (Lippincott-Raven: Atlanta, GA, 1997).

13. Kelley JL, Burke TW, Tornos C, et al. Minimally invasive vulvar carcinoma: an indication for conservative surgical therapy. *Gynecol Oncol* 1992;**44**:240–4.

14. Burke TW, Levenback C, Coleman RL, et al. Surgical therapy of T1 and T2 vulvar carcinoma: further experience with radical wide excision and selective inguinal lymphadenectomy. *Gynecol Oncol* 1995;**57**:215–20.

15. Berman ML, Soper JT, Creasman WT, et al. Conservative surgical management of superficially invasive stage I vulvar carcinoma. *Gynecol Oncol* 1989;**35**:352–7.

16. Hacker NF, Berek JS, Lagasse LD, et al. Individualization of treatment for stage I squamous cell vulvar carcinoma. *Obstet Gynecol* 1984;**63**:155–62.

17. Cherry C, Glucksmann A. Lymphatic embolism and lymph node metastasis in cancers of vulva and of uterine cervix. *Cancer* 1955;**8**:564.

18. Levenback C, Morris M, Burke TW, et al. Groin dissection practices among gynecologic oncologists treating early vulvar cancer. *Gynecol Oncol* 1996;**62**:73–7.

19. Plentl AA, Friedman EA. Clinical significance of the vulvar lymphatics. In: *Lymphatic System of Female Genitalia* (W. B. Saunders: Philadelphia, PA, 1971), 27–50.

20. Stehman FB, Bundy BN, Thomas G, et al. Groin dissection versus groin radiation in carcinoma of the vulva: a Gynecologic Oncology Group study. *Int J Radiat Oncol Biol Phys* 1992;**24**:389–96.

21. Cabanas RM. An approach for the treatment of penile carcinoma. *Cancer* 1977;**39**:456–66.

22. DiSaia PJ, Creasman WT, Rich WM. An alternate approach to early cancer of the vulva. *Am J Obstet Gynecol* 1979;**133**:825–32.

23. Rouzier R, Haddad B, Dubernard G, et al. Inguinofemoral dissection for carcinoma of the vulva: effect of modifications of extent and technique on morbidity and survival. *J Am Coll Surg* 2003;**196**:442–50.

24. Plentl AA, Friedman EA. Lymphatics of the cervix uteri. In: Plentl AA, Friedman EA, eds, *Lymphatic System of Female Genitalia* (WB Saunders: Philadelphia, 1971) 75–115.

25. DiSaia P. Invasive cancer of the vulva. In: DiSaia P, Creasman WT, eds, *Clinical Gynecologic Oncology* (Mosby: St Louis, MO, 2002).

26. Doherty M. Clinical anatomy of the pelvis. In: Copeland L, ed, *Textbook of Gynecology* (WB Saunders: Philadelphia, PA, 1993), 48–84.

2c LYMPHATICS OF THE CERVIX

ROBERT COLEMAN AND CHARLES LEVENBACK

Although the uterine cervix and the uterine corpus differ anatomically and functionally, their respective lymphatic systems are similar. The mucosa, muscularis, and serosa have distinct lymphatic flow, but within each layer, flow between the cervix and the corpus is continuous. We have chosen to discuss the uterine cervix and uterine corpus separately given that tumors arising in the cervix are treated differently from tumors arising in the corpus. Understanding and exploitation of the normal lymphatic anatomy of the uterine cervix has led to refinement and individualization of treatment for the diseased cervix. Further elucidation of how disease affects the lymphatic framework of the cervix and lymphangiogenic processes will be important in clarifying the natural history of cervical cancer and increasing our therapeutic acumen.

TOPOGRAPHIC ANATOMY OF THE CERVIX

Anatomically, the cervix is defined as the region of the uterus from the isthmus to its vaginal termination. Depending on a woman's age and on uterine and cervical factors, the size of the cervix varies with respect to the size of the corpus.[1] In general, the cervix ranges from 2 to 4 cm in length in the nulligravid woman. It is connected to the vagina through an oblique fibrous attachment where approximately one-third of the anterior wall and approximately one-half of the posterior wall are exposed to the vagina (infravaginal cervix)[2] (Figure 2c.1). The vaginal portion, or exocervix, is convex. Centrally located within the

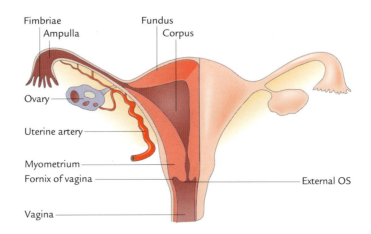

Figure 2c.1 Topographic anatomy of the cervix.

exocervix is the external cervical os. The size of this opening to the uterus varies depending on a woman's age and history of parturition. Proximal to the external os is the elliptical endocervical canal, which terminates at the internal cervical os. Here the cervix joins the uterine isthmus. Anteriorly and posteriorly, the supravaginal cervix is covered by the parietal peritoneum.

The cervix is comprised of fibrous, elastic, and smooth muscular tissue. It is more fibrous than the corpus, with smooth muscle comprising just 15% of the body of the cervix, primarily at the endocervix. It is lined by columnar and squamous epithelium. The endocervix is lined by a single layer of mucin-producing columnar epithelium, which also lines the many endocervical glands. In this respect, the mucin-producing apparatus is not truly glandular but is a complex infolding of the mucosal surface. The distal extent of this mucosa joins stratified, nonkeratinizing squamous epithelium on or near the exocervix. The location of this abrupt transformation is variable and changes continuously during the reproductive years, responding to the lower vaginal pH after puberty.[3] In this process, columnar epithelium undergoes metaplastic change to become more resilient squamous epithelium. It is in this transformation zone that most preinvasive and invasive cervical lesions arise. Distally, the exocervical tissue is continuous with the vaginal epithelium.

The paired uterosacral and cardinal ligaments primarily support the cervix and uterus. The uterosacral ligaments attach at the base of the uterus and run in the rectouterine peritoneal folds to the sacrum. The cardinal ligaments are thickened bands of fibrous tissue in continuation with the endopelvic fascia that extend to the lateral pelvic sidewall (Figure 2c.2). Within these bands also run the nerves and vessels to the cervix and pelvic viscera.

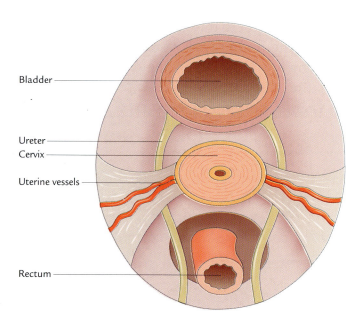

Figure 2c.2   The cervix is supported by the cardinal and uterosacral ligaments, which blend with the fascia of the pelvic diaphragm.

TOPOGRAPHIC ANATOMY OF THE CERVICAL LYMPHATICS

The lymphatic vessels of the endocervical mucosa are found immediately below the cuboidal/columnar glandular epithelium and are irregular in their arrangement. The fragile individual vessels coalesce to form channels, which flow out from the mucosa within the plicae palmatae, generally perpendicular to the axis of the cervical canal. Interfacing with the stroma, the channels flatten and angle to run parallel with the endocervical canal, where they combine further to make larger channels. Ultimately, these vessels converge upon intermediate trunks located within the stromal vasculature. Within the cervical stroma, a dense and regular lattice of lymphatic vessels is found. Near the mucosal surface, lymphatics grossly outnumber vascular channels and seemingly bear no consistent relationship with blood vessels or each other. Circumferentially, as these channels coalesce into larger trunks, they course more regularly with the cervical veins, often surrounding them to the serosa. A small number of reports have documented the existence of a valvular system within stromal lymphatics that prevents retrograde flow in all but disease states.

When the stromal lymphatics reach the serosa, they interface through a series of lacunae, which go on to invest the entire corpus.[4] These major efferent systems coalesce in the cervix to form three dominant extravisceral trunks (anterior, lateral, and posterior). It should be noted that these cervical lymphatic vessels often share terminal nodes with other sites, such as the uterine corpus and the vagina. However, it is relevant that there is little intermixing of lymph; rather, separate lymphatic trunks from these sites run in parallel to common basins and particular terminal nodes. Valves within these trunks also prevent retrograde flow under normal conditions.

Lateral trunk

The largest and most significant pathway of the extravisceral cervical drainage comes from the lateral trunk. There are three branches within this trunk, each of which drains into specific nodal basins within the pelvis (Figure 2c.3). The upper branches of the lateral trunk are two to three large vessels that course from the cervical serosa cephalad and anterior along the path of the uterine vessels, crossing over the ureter and obliterated umbilical artery and coming to rest in the interiliac nodal basin at the bifurcation of the external and internal iliac vessels. The lateral-trunk drainage is considered the dominant drainage of the cervix and was referred to by Leveuf and Godard as 'la voie principale'.[5] The large node in this location is very consistent clinically; however, in its absence, a secondary node is often found in the common iliac chain. On the right, this secondary node is often located on the common iliac vein; on the left, it can be found between the iliopsoas muscle and common iliac artery.

The path of the upper branches of the lateral trunk to the iliac nodes can be interrupted by small parametrial lymph nodes. These lymph nodes are difficult to study. They can easily be overlooked in cadaver studies. In vivo, they are not seen during radical hysterectomy. They are very close to the cervix and therefore are not imaged well on lymphoscintigraphy because of the large amount of residual radioactivity in the cervix. They are not seen well on blue dye studies either, again because of their small size, their proximity to the cervix, and the fact that they are not seen on dissection.

The equally important middle branches of the lateral trunk serve as a dominant pathway to the obturator lymph nodes, also referred to by some as the posterior interiliac nodes. The course of the lymph in this case is along the middle cardinal ligament to the posterior aspect of the internal iliac vessel.

Arising from the lateral dorsal cervix are the lower branches of the lateral trunk. Some of these pass posteriorly around the ureter and course either dorsally to the uterosacral ligament, terminating in the inferior gluteal nodes, or cephalad and ventrally, terminating in the superior gluteal nodes. Still others course posteriorly along the sacral hollow, terminating in the sacral and subaortic nodes directly.

The lower branches of the lateral trunk serve as a pathway to the superior and inferior gluteal lymph nodes. This pathway is described in the classic, cadaver-based anatomic studies. Clinical reports rarely comment on these lymph nodes, and gluteal nodes appear to be a rare site for metastatic disease. The lower branches of the lateral trunk continue on towards the presacral (subaortic) lymph nodes, as described below.

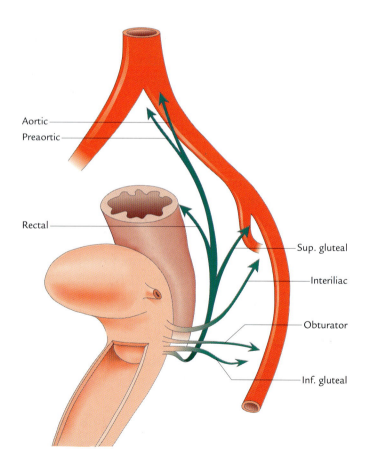

Figure 2c.3　The dominant lateral lymphatic trunk drains into several lower pelvic nodal basins. (Modified from Plentl and Friedman[6]).

Posterior trunk

The posterior collecting trunk primarily drains towards the subaortic nodal basin. This trunk arises from the posterior cervix and courses along the uterosacral ligament to the lateral rectal fascia, continuing anteriorly over the sacral promontory or posteriorly to the superior rectal nodes (Figure 2c.4). Direct drainage to the aortic nodes can be demonstrated in vessels from this trunk, which travel with the ureter to the pelvic brim, where they diverge into the common iliac, subaortic, and aortic nodal basins.

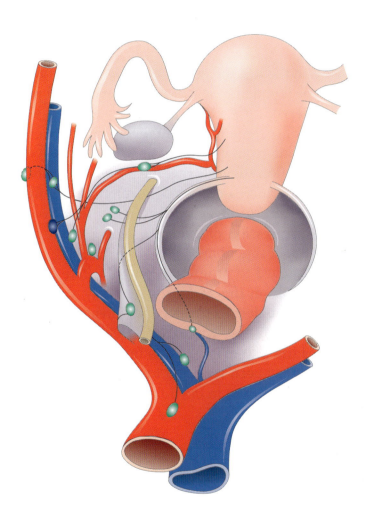

Figure 2c.4   The posterior lymphatic trunk courses along the uterosacral ligament to drain into the common iliac, subaortic, aortic, and superior gluteal nodes. A blue lymph node is shown at a common location to find sentinel lymph nodes in patients with cervical cancer. Sentinel nodes may also be found in obdurator, common iliac, presacral, and para-aortic sites. (Modified from Plenty and Friedman[6]).

Anterior trunk

The anterior trunk leaves the anterior cervix and courses along the posterior surface of the bladder to the superior vesical artery. From there it travels to the obliterated umbilical vessel and terminates in the distal interiliac nodal basins anteriorly. Separate but parallel vessels run along the cardinal ligament, where they meet without intermixing with the lateral trunk and drain into that trunk's distribution.

THE NATURAL HISTORY OF CERVIX CANCER RELEVANT TO ITS LYMPHATIC ANATOMY

Most cancers arising in the uterine cervix are carcinomas of its epithelium. The predominant histologic subtype is squamous; however, an increased proportion of adenocarcinoma has recently been observed.[7] Cervical carcinomas are believed to develop in most cases from a preinvasive lesion, carcinoma in situ, over a number of years. The molecular events driving the transformation from carcinoma in situ to invasive cancer are not well known. However, recent information suggests that the presence of human papillomavirus and high viral load place patients at increased risk of developing cervical cancer.[8] Most certainly, the shift from carcinoma in situ to invasive cancer is a result of the accumulation of genetic errors such as altered expression of the *FHIT* gene and the interaction of human papillomanvirus DNA with the host genome.[9–11]

Cervical cancer is believed to progress through a state of microscopic invasion into the stroma and radial growth on the surface. Ultimately, a locus is formed that, in general, grows locally to invade the deeper stroma and, later, the paracervical and parametrial tissues. If left untreated, the disease will expand through these tissues to involve the lateral pelvic side wall. In addition, it may grow to involve the bladder, rectum, or both. Cancer arising from the cervix has been reported to extend into the uterine corpus in 10–30% of cases and into the uterine adnexa in 0.5–1.6% of cases. Lateral spread is the rule; however,

Table 2c.1 Likelihood of lymph node metastases in patients with early-stage cervical cancer.

Stage	% of patients with metastases
IA_1	0.15
IA_2	1.13
IB_1	16
IB_2	32
IIA	25
IIB	43

as many as 17% of patients with early-stage cervix cancer have lymph node metastases.[12] The likelihood of nodal involvement by disease stage among patients with early-stage disease is shown in Table 2c.1. The pelvic nodes, as a group, are the most commonly involved nodes. It is very uncommon to find isolated para-aortic lymphatic disease in the absence of metastatic pelvic disease.[12] This observation has led to the consensus determination that lymphatic spread occurs in a sequential pattern from the external iliac to common iliac to aortic lymph nodes. The lymphatic anatomy of the cervix suggests that an individual patient could have a common iliac sentinel lymph node metastasis in the absences of an external iliac metastasis; however, this clinical observation is very rare.

Hematogenous spread of disease is generally a finding associated with late presentation and most commonly involves the lungs, bone, intra-abdominal viscera, or distal lymphatics.[13] Variant cell types, such as neuroendocrine or glassy cell carcinoma, may be associated with distant disease in the absence of local proliferation. Current therapy for these variants typically involves multimodality strategies designed to address the tumor's potential for local and distant metastasis.[14]

SUMMARY

Lymphatic anatomy of the cervix is surprisingly complex. Pelvic lymph nodes actually refer to several nodal basins immediately adjacent to one another. Lymphatic mapping studies have the potential to help understand the clinical significance, if any, of the various anatomic variations.

REFERENCES

1. Bartoli JM, Moulin G, Delannoy L, et al. The normal uterus on magnetic resonance imaging and variations associated with the hormonal state. *Surg Radiol Anat* 1991;**13**:213–20.
2. Ferenczy A, Wright T. Anatomy and histology of the cervix. In: *Blaustein's Pathology of the Female Genital Tract* Kurman RK, ed, (Springer-Verlag: New York, 1994) 185–201.
3. Singer A. The uterine cervix from adolescence to the menopause. *Br J Obstet Gynaecol* 1975;**82**:81–99.
4. Plentl AA, Friedman EA. Lymphatics of the cervix uteri. In: *Lymphatic System of Female Genitalia* (WB Saunders: Philadelphia, PA, 1971) 75–115.
5. Leveuf J, Godard H. Les lymphatiques de l'utérus. *Rev Chir* 1923;**3**:219–48.
6. Plentl AA, Friedman EA. Lymphatics of the cervix uteri. In: *Lymphatic System of Female Genitalia* (WB Saunders: Philadelphia, 1971) 75–115.
7. Zaino RJ. Glandular lesions of the uterine cervix. *Mod Pathol* 2000;**13**:261–74.
8. Josefsson AM, Magnusson PK, Ylitalo N, et al. Viral load of human papilloma virus 16 as a determinant for development of cervical carcinoma in situ: a nested case-control study. *Lancet* 2000;**355**:2189–93.

48

9. Park TW, Fujiwara H, Wright TC. Molecular biology of cervical cancer and its precursors. *Cancer* 1995;**76**(10 Suppl):1902–13.

10. Muller CY, O'Boyle JD, Fong KM, et al. Abnormalities of fragile histidine triad genomic and complementary DNAs in cervical cancer: association with human papillomavirus type. *J Natl Cancer Inst* 1998;**90**:433–9.

11. Wistuba II, et al. Deletions of chromosome 3p are frequent and early events in the pathogenesis of uterine cervical carcinoma. *Cancer Res* 1997;**57**:3154–8.

12. Hopkins MP, Morley GW. Stage IB squamous cell cancer of the cervix: clinicopathologic features related to survival. *Am J Obstet Gynecol* 1991;**164**:1520–7.

13. Delgado G, et al. A prospective surgical pathological study of stage I squamous carcinoma of the cervix: a Gynecologic Oncology Group study. *Gynecol Oncol* 1989;**36**:314–20.

14. Lagasse LD, et al. Results and complications of operative staging in cervical cancer: experiences of the Gynecologic Oncology Group. *Gynecol Oncol* 1980;**9**:90–8.

2d LYMPHATICS OF THE CORPUS UTERI

ATE VAN DER ZEE

INTRODUCTION

Understanding the pattern of lymphatic spread of endometrial cancer is crucial to predicting prognosis and designing a rational therapy. The presence of lymph node metastases has a major impact on the prognosis of women with endometrial cancer.[1] Systematic pelvic and aortic lymphadenectomy appears to be the most sensitive way to assess a patient's lymph node status. In addition it has been argued that failure to sample pelvic and para-aortic nodes systematically results in a small, but real, risk of undetected extrauterine metastasis. Instead of a complete systematic pelvic and aortic lymphadenectomy, however, it appears that a selective approach to sampling that includes biopsy from both para-aortic and bilateral pelvic lymphatic zones provides an accurate estimate of true node negativity.[2] Lymphatic mapping of the retroperitoneal nodes that drain the corpus uteri in a patient with endometrial cancer has the potential to increase the effectiveness of a lymphadenectomy and might offer the potential to reduce the amount of dissection required, possibly also resulting in less morbidity for the patient.

Information on the lymphatics of the corpus uteri in general can be obtained from three different types of studies; the first is descriptive anatomic reports in which the lymphatic anatomy is studied with or without previous injection of different types of dyes. A second source of information comprises studies on the distribution of pelvic and para-aortic lymph node metastases in patients with endometrial cancer who underwent pelvic and para-aortic lymphadenectomy. The third and last type of studies are those in which lymphatic mapping by injection of a tracer has been performed in patients with endometrial cancer. In this section on lymphatics of the corpus uteri, the three different types of studies will be discussed.

LYMPHATIC ANATOMY

Most studies on the lymphatic anatomy of the uterus are quite old and go back to the first half of the twentieth century. Our current understanding of the uterine lymphatic bed stems from studies such as those by Kroemer[3] and Reiffenstuhl,[4] who applied ex vivo retrograde filling of the uterine lymphatics with a dye solution. These studies were summarized nicely by Plentl and Friedman in 1971.[5] More recent studies, applying light and electron microscopy, resulted in our current view on uterine lymphatics.

Blackwell and Fraser demonstrated that the endometrial lymphatic bed takes its origin in channels arising just beneath the glandular lining cells.[6] The lymphatic capillaries coalesce in the endometrial stroma to form fine collecting channels in the basalis layer of the endometrium. Near the inner muscle margin, they turn to join with other endometrial collecting lymphatics, forming a network in the deepest portion of the endometrium at its junction with the myometrium, parallel with the uterine lumen. Perpendicular perforating lymph vessels originate from these submyometrial lacunae, and subsequently enter the muscularis directly and form a very regular pattern. New lymph capillaries arise in association with myometrial cells and anastomose freely with perforating efferents on their course toward the serosal surface. As these lymph vessels wend peripherally, they enlarge in diameter and approach the corresponding veins draining the myometrium. In the sharp junction between the muscularis and the serosa, the lymphatic trunks turn acutely to form the 'subserosal network' (Figure 2d.1). This coarse lymphatic mesh forms throughout the interface and drains all the lymph flowing from the more centrally located tissues of endometrium and myometrium. Trunks arising from this network form the collecting channels that drain the uterus extraviscerally. They are joined by the serosal lymphatics, which contribute the third source of lymph from the uterus. This subserosal network is

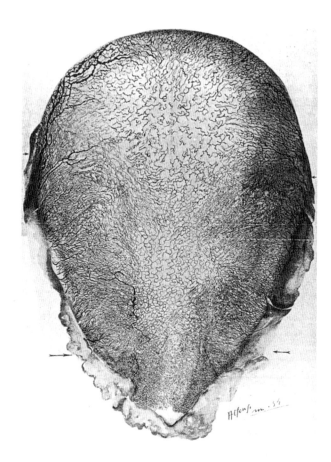

Figure 2d.1 Subserosal network of uterine lymphatics (Modified from Plentl and Friedman[5]).

characterized by a strong confluence of the plexus towards the lateral margins of the uterus. Anastomoses exist between corpus and cervix within the mucosal and muscular layers. The corpus uteri is drained by four well-established channels:

1) Channels draining the fundus uteri in company with the ovarian vessels, ultimately traveling to the level of the lower pole of the kidney and terminating in the aortic nodes in the vicinity of the renal and superior mesenteric arteries.

2) Channels emerging from the lateral edges of the middle and lower parts of the corpus uteri within the folds of the broad ligament, and terminating in the uppermost interiliac nodes. Within the folds of the broad ligament, a longitudinal drainage channel is found, the 'anastomosis of Poirier'. It connects the lymphatic bed of the uterus with that of the cervix with a unidirectional flow from the uterus to the cervix.

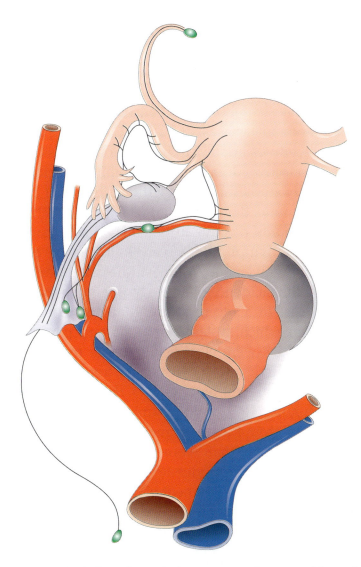

Figure 2d.2 The uterus has multiple lymphatic drainage routes that extend from the groin to just below the renal vessels. (Modified from Plentl and Friedman[5]).

3) Anastomotic channels, especially near the cornua, along the mesosalpinx and tubular bed, terminating, together with the ovarian lymp channels, in the aortic and superior gluteal nodes.

4) Probably least important, lymphatics along the round ligament directed towards the deep femoral nodes (Figure 2d.2).

In summary, from these anatomic studies, the aortic, interiliac, and femoral nodes can be regarded as the primary regional nodes draining the corpus uteri, while indirectly, through lymphatic anastomoses, the external iliac and superior gluteal nodes may also assume this role.

DISTRIBUTION OF PELVIC AND PARA-AORTIC LYMPH NODE METASTASES IN PATIENTS WITH ENDOMETRIAL CANCER

For endometrial cancer, the route of lymphatic spread remains to be clarified, possibly because of a paucity of accurate data on the distribution of lymph node metastases in this malignancy. Most studies in endometrial cancer have shown conflicting results on the distribution of lymph node metastases, and these conflicting data are especially ascribable to different surgical procedures applied to lymph node assessment, such as sampling of only enlarged nodes and selective, or systematic, lymphadenectomy.

Mariani et al recently studied patients with endometrial cancer with and without cervical involvement and found that the external iliac and obturator lymph nodes were the pelvic sites most commonly positive in patients with tumors confined to the uterine corpus, while external iliac lymph nodes were followed by common iliac lymph nodes in patients with cervical involvement.[7] Many studies in endometrial cancer have also shown conflicting results on the incidence of aortic lymph node metastasis with or without pelvic lymph node metastasis. In a recent study, Matsumoto et al reported on node-positive endometrial cancers in which systematic pelvic and para-aortic lymphadenectomy was performed.[8] Lymph nodes were classified into the five subgroups: aortic lymph nodes above the inferior mesenteric artery (IMA) (A1), aortic lymph nodes below the IMA (A2), the common iliac and sacral lymph nodes (P1), the internal and external iliac lymph nodes and obturator lymph nodes (P2), and the suprainguinal lymph nodes (P3). In endometrial cancer, nodes in the subgroups A1, A2, and P2 were involved at high rates, while metastases to P2 were more frequent than A1 or A2. The relatively high prevalence of metastasis at both pelvic and aortic lymph nodes (67%) is in keeping with previous studies documenting that the incidence of involvement of both pelvic and aortic lymph nodes is 27–80% in endometrial cancer.[1,2,9–12] Aortic lymph node metastases were also analyzed in relation to the positivity of P1, a subgroup including the common iliac nodes, which could be assumed to be affected when aortic lymph node metastases occur by spreading from pelvic nodes. Although aortic lymph node metastases were associated with P1 positivity in endometrial cancer, in 7% of cases, aortic lymph node involvement alone was observed. Comparable figures on aortic lymph node metastases in endometrial cancer have been reported by others.[1,2,9–12]

From this summary of the literature on the distribution of lymph node metastases in endometrial cancer, it appears that endometrial cancer can directly metastasize to both pelvic and aortic lymph nodes, with pelvic lymph node metastases being predominant.

SENTINEL NODE DETECTION IN ENDOMETRIAL CANCER

Up to now, three feasibility studies on sentinel node detection in endometrial cancer have been reported. In 1996, Burke et al described a study of intraperitoneal lymphatic mapping of the uterine fundus as a means of identifying target sites for lymph node biopsy during staging laparotomy. In 15 women with high-risk endometrial tumor, isosulfan blue dye was injected at laparotomy into the subserosal myometrium at three sites of the uterine fundus. Lymphatic channels coursing into the broad ligament and along the ovarian vessels were identified from all uteri injected. Deposition of dye into grossly identifiable lymph nodes was seen in 67% of cases, and the locations of these nodes included aortic sites (all above the inferior mesenteric artery), and common iliac and pelvic sites. It appeared from this study that, indeed, the lymphatic network draining the uterus is complex and involves both pelvic and para-aortic nodes.[13] In 2002, two studies on lymphatic mapping were reported. Holub et al showed the feasibility of two intraoperative procedures of lymphatic mapping and sentinel node detection, using a blue dye in 25 surgically staged patients with early-stage endometrial cancer. At laparoscopy, patent blue-V was injected into the subserosal myometrium or cervico-subserosal myometrium. In the majority of patients, a deposition of the blue dye was found in at least one pelvic lymph node.[14] Using a combination of a radioactive tracer and blue dye in 11 patients with early-stage endometrial cancer, Pelosi et al performed laparoscopic sentinel lymph node (SLN) detection during laparoscopy-assisted vaginal hysterectomy with bilateral salpingo-oophorectomy and bilateral systematic pelvic lymphadenectomy. Both the radioactive tracer and blue dye were injected in the cervix. The same SLN locations detected with the gamma scintiprobe were observed at laparoscopy after patent blue dye injection.[15]

REFERENCES

1. Morrow CP, Bundy BN, Kurman RJ, et al. Relationship between surgical-pathological risk factors and outcome in clinical stage I and II carcinoma of the endometrium: a Gynecologic Oncology Group study. *Gynecol Oncol* 1991;**40**:55–65.
2. Chuang L, Burke TW, Tornos C, et al. Staging laparotomy for endometrial carcinoma: assessment of retroperitoneal lymph nodes. *Gynecol Oncol* 1995;**58**:189–93.

3. Kroemer P. Die Lymphorgane der weiblichen Genitalien und ihre Veranderungen bei maligne Erkrankugen des Uterus. *Arch Gynak* 1904;**73**:57.

4. Reiffenstuhl G. *Das Lymphsystem des weiblichen Genitale.* (Urban & Schwarzenberg: Munchen, 1957).

5. Plentl AA, Friedman EA. Lymphatics of the cervix uteri. In: *Lymphatic System of Female Genitalia.* (WB Saunders: Philadelphia, PA, 1971) 75–115.

6. Blackwell PM, Fraser IS. Superficial lymphatics in the functional zone of normal human endometrium. *Microvasc Res* 1981;**21**:142–52.

7. Mariani A, Webb MJ, Keeney GL, et al. Routes of lymphatic spread: a study of 112 consecutive patients with endometrial cancer. *Gynecol Oncol* 2001;**81**:100–4.

8. Matsumoto K, Yoshikawa H, Yasugi T, et al. Distinct lymphatic spread of endometrial carcinoma in comparison with cervical and ovarian carcinomas. *Cancer Lett* 2002;**180**:83–9.

9. Ayhan A, Yarali H, Urman B, et al. Lymph node metastasis in early endometrium cancer. *Aust N Z J Obstet Gynaecol* 1989;**29**(3 Pt 2):332–5.

10. Larson DM, Johnson KK. Pelvic and para-aortic lymphadenectomy for surgical staging of high-risk endometrioid adenocarcinoma of the endometrium. *Gynecol Oncol* 1993;**51**:345–8.

11. Yokoyama Y, Maruyama H, Sato S, et al. Indispensability of pelvic and paraaortic lymphadenectomy in endometrial cancers. *Gynecol Oncol* 1997;**64**:411–17.

12. Hirahatake K, Hareyama H, Sakuragi N, et al. A clinical and pathologic study of para-aortic lymph node metastasis in endometrial carcinoma. *J Surg Oncol* 1997;**65**:82–7.

13. Burke TW, Levenback C, Tornos C, et al. Intraabdominal lymphatic mapping to direct selective pelvic and paraaortic lymphadenectomy in women with high-risk endometrial cancers: results of a pilot study. *Gynecol Oncol* 1996;**62**:169–73.

14. Holub Z, Jabor A, Kliment L. Comparison of two procedures for sentinel lymph node detection in patients with endometrial cancer: a pilot study. *Eur J Gynaecol Oncol* 2002;**23**:53–7.

15. Pelosi E, Arena V, Baudino B, et al. Preliminary study of sentinel node identification with 99mTc colloid and blue dye in patients with endometrial cancer. *Tumori* 2002;**88**:S9–S10.

2e LYMPHATICS OF THE OVARY

ATE VAN DER ZEE

INTRODUCTION

In contrast to the other major gynecologic malignancies, information on the lymphatics of the ovary can be obtained from only two different types of studies; first, descriptive anatomy reports in which the lymphatic anatomy is studied with or without previous injection of different types of dyes, and, second, studies on the distribution of pelvic and aortic lymph node metastases in patients with ovarian cancer who underwent pelvic and aortic lymph node evaluation. Studies are not available in which lymphatic mapping by injection of a tracer has been performed in patients with ovarian cancer. This lack of studies on lymphatic mapping may well be due to the fact that lymphogenous pathways are not always of primary relevance in the dissemination of ovarian cancers. The most common and earliest mode of dissemination is by exfoliation of cells that implant along the surfaces of the peritoneal cavity. However, in 1985, the International Federation of Gynecologists and Obstetricians (FIGO) modified the staging for ovarian cancer, in part to reflect the prognostic significance of metastatic spread to the pelvic or para-aortic lymph nodes.[1] Especially in patients with disease macroscopically confined to one of the ovaries, survival decreases significantly when retroperitoneal extension is found, thereby emphasizing the need for proper evaluation of the lymph nodes, and consequently justifying more aggressive adjunctive therapy when positive nodes are found.[2]

LYMPHATIC ANATOMY

The tunica albuginea of the ovary is essentially devoid of lymphatics, while the parenchymal lymphatics comprise a rich network, whose presence is related to developing follicles. Lymph from the ovary is drained peripherally by six to eight large collecting trunks that leave the ovarian hilus within the mesovarium to form the subovarian plexus, which is composed of efferent trunks from the uterine corpus, fallopian tube, and ovary. Mixing of lymph that has originated from each organ does occur. Efferent vessels from this plexus drain in a cephalad direction along with the ovarian blood vessels to terminate in the aortic nodes. In about 25% of women, a collateral trunk exists which bypasses the subovarian plexus. It reaches the pelvic wall within the folds of the broad ligament, terminating in the uppermost interiliac nodes.[3]

DISTRIBUTION OF PELVIC AND AORTIC LYMPH NODE METASTASIS IN PATIENTS WITH OVARIAN CANCER

When one looks at ovarian cancer, pelvic and aortic nodes could also be primary and sentinel ones, in view of the frequent observations of pelvic and aortic lymph node metastasis alone in patients with ovarian cancer. In a recent study by Matsumoto et al, in which systematic pelvic and aortic lymph node dissection was performed, the incidence of aortic lymph node metastasis alone in node-positive ovarian cancer patients (all FIGO stages) was 21%,[4] a figure which is consistent with figures previously reported (15–55%).[5–8] Overall, these data show that direct metastasis to the aortic lymph nodes frequently occurs in ovarian cancer. The group of Matsumoto also showed that metastasis at both pelvic and aortic lymph nodes is common in ovarian cancer, again in keeping with previous studies in ovarian cancer. However, the incidence of aortic lymph node metastasis was not related to incidence of positive common iliac and sacral nodes, a subgroup which could be assumed to be affected when aortic lymph node metastasis spreading from pelvic nodes occurs. In combination with an incidence of pelvic lymph node metastasis alone in patients with ovarian cancer of 17%, these data clearly indicate two separate ways of lymphatic spread in ovarian cancer.

Therefore, it appears that metastasis in ovarian cancer may take two separate routes; one via the broad ligament to the internal and external iliac and obturator lymph nodes and one via the infundibulopelvic ligament to the aortic lymph nodes (Figure 2e.1).

The pattern of lymphatic spread in ovarian cancer macroscopically confined to one ovary is controversial with respect to whether contralateral lymph node metastases do occur. In a retrospective study in this category of patients, Cass et al found positive pelvic nodes alone in 50%, positive aortic nodes alone in 36%, and both in 14% of cases, while isolated contralateral lymph node metastases were seen in 4%.[9] Comparable low figures have also been reported by others,[10–13] while several studies did not find contralateral metastases.[14,15] Based on the lymphatic anatomy, it is hard to imagine the way of contralateral spread. All the studies that have reported contralateral metastasis were retrospective, and it may well be that a lesion such as occult disease in the ipsilateral ovary has been missed.

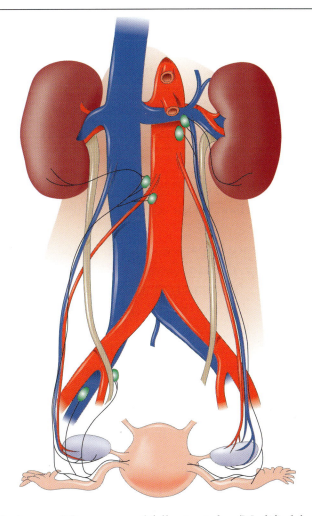

Figure 2e.1 Lymphatic drainage of the ovary and fallopian tube. (Modified from Plentl and Friedman[3]).

SENTINEL NODE DETECTION IN OVARIAN CANCER

As already mentioned in the introduction of this chapter, no data are available on lymphatic mapping in ovarian cancer. Apart from the fact that in ovarian cancer lymphatic spread is not as prominent as intraperitoneal spread, there are several other issues that raise doubts on the possible applicability of lymphatic mapping in ovarian cancer. It seems obvious that the only category of patients with ovarian cancer that might be eligible for sentinel node detection are patients with tumors confined to one or both ovaries. However, even in these patients, it is hard to imagine where in the tumor the tracer should be injected. Perhaps, injection of the tracer somewhere in the hilus of the ovarian tumor is most rational, but it remains to be seen whether this will be representative of the spread of the cancer, hidden somewhere in the pelvic mass. Another issue is that in most patients with a tumor confined to the ovary the only way to establish the diagnosis is removal of the tumor, and after removal it will no longer be possible to perform lymphatic mapping. From these considerations, lymphatic mapping on first sight does not seem to be a promising technique in ovarian cancer.

REFERENCES

1. FIGO, Changes in gynecologic staging by the Internation Federation of Gynecologists and Obstetricians. *Am J Obstet Gynecol* 1990;**162**:610–11.
2. Carnino F, Fuda G, Ciccone G, et al. Significance of lymph node sampling in epithelial carcinoma of the ovary. *Gynecol Oncol* 1997;**65**:467–72.
3. Plentl A, Friedman E. *Lymphatic System of the Female Genitalia*. Vol. 2. (WB Saunders: Philadelphia, PA, 1971).
4. Matsumoto K, Yoshikawa H, Yasugi T, et al. Distinct lymphatic spread of endometrial carcinoma in comparison with cervical and ovarian carcinomas. *Cancer Letters* 2002;**180**:83–9.
5. Chen SS, Lee L. Incidence of para-aortic and pelvic lymph node metastases in epithelial carcinoma of the ovary. *Gynecol Oncol* 1983;**16**:95–100.
6. Onda T, Yoshikawa H, Yokota H, et al. Assessment of metastases to aortic and pelvic lymph nodes in epithelial ovarian carcinoma. A proposal for essential sites for lymph node biopsy. *Cancer* 1996;**78**:803–8.
7. Sakai K, Kamura T, Hirakawa T, et al. Relationship between pelvic lymph node involvement and other disease sites in patients with ovarian cancer. *Gynecol Oncol* 1997;**65**:164–8.
8. Tsumura N, Sakuragi N, Hareyama H, et al. Distribution pattern and risk factors of pelvic and para-aortic lymph node metastasis in epithelial ovarian carcinoma. *Int J Cancer* 1998;**79**:526–30.
9. Cass I, Li AJ, Runowicz CD, et al. Pattern of lymph node metastases in clinically unilateral stage I invasive epithelial ovarian carcinomas. *Gynecol Oncol* 2001;**80**:56–61.
10. Wu P, Qu J, Lang J, et al. Lymph node metastasis of ovarian cancer: a preliminary survey of 74 cases of lymphadenectomy. *Am J Obstet Gynecol* 1986;**155**:1103–8.
11. Petru E, Lahousen M, Tamussino K, et al. Lymphadenectomy in stage I ovarian cancer. *Am J Obstet Gynecol* 1994;**170**:656–62.
12. Onda T, Yoshikawa H, Yasugi T, et al. Patients with ovarian carcinoma upstaged to stage III after systematic lymphadenectomy have similar survival to stage I/II patients and superior survival to other stage III patients. *Cancer* 1998;**83**:1555–60.
13. Walter AJ, Magrina JF. Contralateral pelvic and aortic lymph node metastasis in clinical stage I epithelial ovarian cancer. *Gynecol Oncol* 1999;**74**:128–9.
14. Burghardt E, Girardi F, Lahousen M, et al. Patterns of pelvic and paraaortic lymph node involvement in ovarian cancer. *Gynecol Oncol* 1991;**40**:103–6.
15. Benedetti Panici P, Greggi S, Maneschi F, et al. Anatomical and pathological study of retroperitoneal nodes in epithelial ovarian cancer. *Gynecol Oncol* 1993;**51**:150–4.

2f LYMPHATIC ANATOMY OF THE BREAST AND AXILLA

JAMES V. FIORICA

Lymphatic mapping of the breast is altering the long-standing approach to the breast cancer treatment model, radical mastectomy with complete axillary lymphadenectomy. It is a dramatic departure from Halsted's modality of 100 years ago.[1] The breast lies within the superficial fascia of the anterior thoracic wall. It is situated between the second and sixth ribs and the sternal edge and midaxillary line. The posterior surface of the breast ends abruptly at the chest wall when it reaches the pectoralis major fascia. It is composed of skin, parenchyma, and stroma. The stroma and connective tissue are intertwined with blood vessels, nerves, and lymphatics. Beneath the nipples are 5–10 milk ducts which connect to 5–10 additional ducts, each draining an individual breast lobe. Each lobe is composed of 20–40 lobules, which in turn connect to 10–100 tubulosaccular units called alveoli. The subcutaneous connective tissue surrounds glands and extends as septa between the lobes and lobules, providing support for the glandular elements. Cooper's ligaments are suspensory structures which insert perpendicular to the dermis.

The pectoralis major muscle is a fan-shaped muscle with two divisions. The clavicular division originates from the clavicle and can be easily distinguished from the larger costosternal division that originates from the sternum and costal cartilage of ribs 2–6. These fibers converge on the greater tubercle of the humerus. The pectoralis minor muscle is located beneath the pectoralis major muscle and arises from the external surface of ribs 2–5. The posterior suspensory ligaments extend from the deep surface of the breast to the deep pectoral fascia. The subscapular muscle arises from the first rib near the costochondral junction and extends laterally to insert on the inferior surface of the clavicle.

The axillary sheath extends from the neck to the axilla and is surrounded by a layer of fascia. This sheath contains the great vessels and nerves of the upper extremities. The axillary artery is divided into three parts. The first segment, located medial to the pectoralis minor muscle, has the supreme thoracic branch. This segment supplies the 1st and 2nd intercostal spaces. The second segment, located posterior to the pectoralis minor muscle, contains the thoracoacromial trunk and the lateral thoracic artery branches. Located lateral to the pectoralis minor muscle is the third segment of the axillary artery. It has three branches, which are the anterior and posterior humoral circumflex arteries and the subscapular artery. The largest of the axillary branches is this subscapular artery. This artery branches into the subscapular circumflex and the thoracodorsal arteries, which are associated with the central and subscapular lymph nodes, which are described in more detail later in this paper.

The internal mammary artery medially (65%) and the lateral thoracic artery (35%) supply blood to the breast (Figure 2f.1). The cephalic vein serves as a landmark separating the pectoralis major muscle from the deltoid muscle. The vein travels through the deltopectoral triangle and pierces the clavipectoral fascia, joining the axillary vein. Branches of the brachial plexus are located throughout the course of the axilla. The long thoracic nerve is located on the medial wall of the axilla, arising in the neck from the fifth, sixth, and seventh roots of the brachial plexus. It innervates the serratus anterior muscle, which permits raising the arm above the shoulder. The intercostobrachial nerve is the lateral cutaneous branch of the second intercostal nerve and the joining of the medial cutaneous nerve of the arm, supplying the skin of the floor of the axilla and the upper medial aspect of the arm.

The lymphatic system of the breast is just as intricate and complicated. The subaerolar lymphatic plexus of Sappey communicates to the vertical lymphatics in a subepithelial and subdermal manner. The unidirectional lymphatics flow from this superficial subaerolar plexus through the lactiferous duct lymphatics to the perilobar and deep subcutaneous lymphatic plexus. This deep lymphatic plexus drains in a centrifugal direction to the axillary nodes (97%) and the internal mammary nodes (3%). The axillary nodes are divided into six groups: *the lateral* (axillary) group lies medial and posterior to the axillary vein (4–6 nodes), the *external mammary group* (anterior or pectoral) lies along the lower border of the pectoralis minor muscle adjacent to the lateral thoracic vessels (4–5 nodes), the *subscapular* (posterior) group lies along the posterior wall of the axilla at the lateral border of the scapula (6–7 nodes), and the *central* group is embedded in the fat of the axilla behind the pectoralis minor muscle and is the common shallow palpable group of nodes (3–4 nodes). The *apical* (subclavicular) nodes are located at the upper border of the pectoralis minor muscle and receive lymph from all areas (6–12 nodes). Two additional pathways are the transpectoral and the retropectoral (Rotter's nodes). Rotter's interpectoral group is located between the pectoralis major and minor muscles (1–4 nodes) and passes to the central and apical nodes directly. Prepectoral nodes refer to single lymph nodes, which are found in the subcutaneous tissue within the breast (Figure 2f.2).

The internal mammary nodes are located in the retrosternal interspaces within 2 cm of the sternal margin and transverse the internal mammary vessels. The right internal mammary nodes enter the internal mammary lymphatic trunk, which terminates in the subclavicular nodal group. The left internal mammary chain enters the main thoracic duct.[2]

The level of nodes is often described as level I, II, or III in relationship to the pectoralis minor muscle. Nodal tissue lateral to the minor muscle is known as level I (external mammary, lateral, and subscapular). Those lymphatics beneath the muscle are level II (central ± subscapular), and the lymph nodes on the medial edge of the pectoralis minor muscle are known as level III (apical) lymph nodes. During the standard dissection, level I and a portion of level II nodes are removed[3] (Table 2f.1).

Advocates of the axillary dissection contend that this method renders regional control of axillary disease. Since the time of Halsted, the status of the regional nodal basin has remained the single most important variable in predicting prognosis.[4] Recent thinking supports the idea that microscopic disease may be cured with adjuvant chemotherapy with or

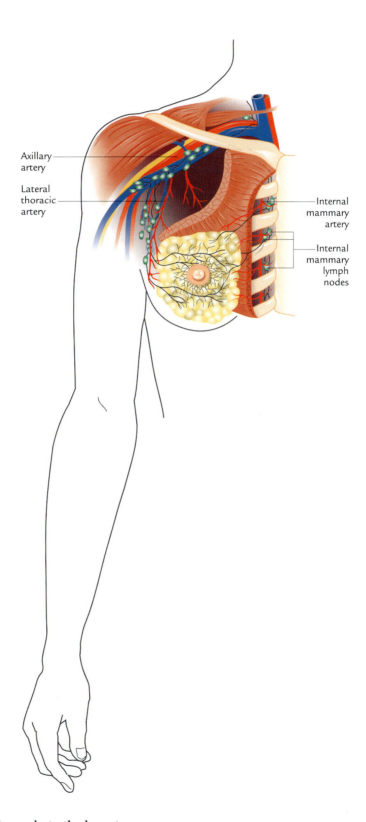

Axillary artery

Lateral thoracic artery

Internal mammary artery

Internal mammary lymph nodes

Figure 2f.1 Primary blood supply to the breast.

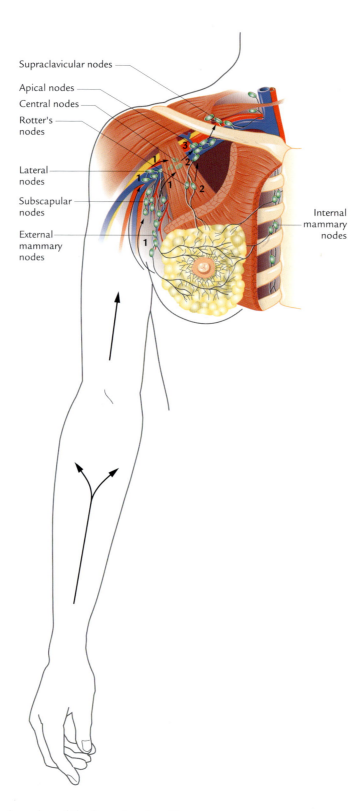

Figure 2f.2   Primary lymph nodes of the breast and axilla.

Table 2f.1 Classification of lymph nodes draining the breast.

Nodal group	Anatomic name	Level	Number of nodes
Axillary	External mammary	I	4–5
	Subscapular	I	6–7
	Lateral	I	4–6
	Central	II	3–4
	Rotter's	II	1–4
	Apical	III	6–12
Internal mammary		–	6–8
Prepectoral nodes		–	1
Deltopectoral		–	1–2
Supraclavicular	(Stage IV)	–	2–3

without node dissection. Some physicians advocate abandoning the axillary lymph node dissection. The development of intraoperative lymphatic mapping and selective lymphadenectomy has permitted the mapping of lymphatic flow from the primary tumor and the identification of the sentinel lymph node (SLN) in the regional basin.

SLN biopsy for breast cancer may obviate the need for routine axillary node dissections in most node-negative patients and still provide prognostic information to the patient and clinician. The assignment of levels I, II, and III was relatively arbitrary and has led to a high (15%) prevalence of skip metastasis.[5] When lymphatic mapping is performed in patients with upper outer quadrant tumors, about 10–15% drain to level II axillary nodes.[6] With lymphatic mapping, variations of breast lymph drainage have been apparent. Direct lymphatic drainage from primary sites has been noted to level II and III axillary nodes, subclavian nodes, and supraclavicular nodes. More accurate staging can improve survival by identifying patients who will gain with either the surgical procedure itself (complete dissection) or the accompanying adjuvant therapy.[7] Additionally, sentinel node biopsy will reduce complications from more extensive surgical procedures or adjuvant therapies. If the women do have micrometastasis in the supraclavicular nodes, they are classified as having stage IV disease.

With proper injection techniques and timing, certain anatomic landmarks are helpful for identifying the sentinel node. If one draws a line from the lateral border of the pectoralis major muscle, and another at the lateral border for the latissimus dorsi muscle in the axilla, these lines would outline the outer borders of the axillary limits for dissection. A tangential line is drawn at the axillary hairline in a perpendicular, anterior to posterior direction. Another line can then be drawn through the axis of the axilla, through the center point of the hairline. The intersecting lines mark the center of a 5-cm circle on the axilla. Ninety-four percent of the SLNs are within this circle. The remaining 6% are in the level II location (Figure 2f.3). Once the SLN is identified on the skin, an accurate incision may be made,

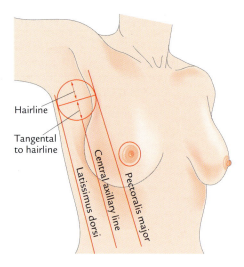

Figure 2f.3 Location of sentinel lymph nodes of the axilla.

overlying the area of highest activity with the gamma probe. Internally, the anatomic land-marks are the central axillary vein and the third branch of the intercostal nerve beneath the clavipectoral fascia. The vein may be found easily, and when the nerve crosses over the vein, four quadrants are defined within the circle described above. The node is considered a SLN if it is blue, or has a blue-stained afferent lymphatic vessel leading to it. In addition, the node is sentinel if it has an in vivo radioactivity (radioactivity in the SLN/neighboring non-SLN) of 3:1 or an ex vivo activity of 10:1.[8]

The mapping techniques vary slightly from center to center. However, the results have attained similar high success rates in skilled hands. Sensitivity and diagnostic accuracy rates have been greater than 95%, with false-negative (skip) rates of 0–10%. These results suggest that lymphatic mapping has the potential to change the standards for surgical management of breast cancer.[9]

REFERENCES

1. Chua B, Ung O, Boyages J. Competing considerations in regional nodal treatment for early breast cancer. *Breast J* 2002;**8**:15–22.
2. Romrell L, Bland K. Anatomy of the breast, axilla, chest wall, and related metastatic sites. In: Bland K, Copeland E, eds, *The Breast. Comprehensive Management of Benign and Malignant Diseases* (W. B. Saunders: Philadelphia, PA, 1991) 17–35.
3. Nathanson SD, Wachna DL, Gilman D, et al. Pathways of lymphatic drainage from the breast. *Ann Surg Oncol* 2001;**8**:837–43.
4. Kramer WM, Rush BF. Mammary duct proliferation in the elderly. A histopathologic study. *Cancer* 1973;**31**:130–7.

5. Veronesi U, Rilke F, Luini A, et al. Distribution of axillary node metastases by level of invasion. An analysis of 539 cases. *Cancer* 1987;**59**:682–7.

6. Feinstein AR, Sosin DM, Wells CK. The Will Rogers phenomenon. Stage migration and new diagnostic techniques as a source of misleading statistics for survival in cancer. *N Engl J Med* 1985;**312**:1604–7.

7. Tanis PJ, Nieweg OE, Valdes Olmos RA, et al. Anatomy and physiology of lymphatic drainage of the breast from the perspective of sentinel node biopsy. *J Am Coll Surg* 2001;**192**:399–409.

8. Cox C. Techniques for lymphatic mapping in breast carcinoma. In: Whitman D, Reintgen D, eds, *Radioguided Surgery* (Landes Biosciences: Austin, TX, 1999) 72–82.

9. Reintgen D, Giuliano R, Cox C. Lymphatic mapping and sentinel lymph node biopsy for breast cancer. *Cancer J* 2002;**8**(Suppl 1):S15–S21.

3 MODALITIES OF DETECTION OF SENTINEL NODES IN LYMPHATIC MAPPING

PEDRO T. RAMIREZ AND CHARLES LEVENBACK

INTRODUCTION

The purpose of this chapter is to review the various techniques for preoperative and intra-operative sentinel lymph node identification. A firm understanding of the definition of a sentinel node and technical aspects of lymphatic mapping will lead to increased success in the operating room and improved outcomes for patients.

WHAT IS A SENTINEL NODE?

The definition of a sentinel node proposed by Morton in 1992[1] is 'the first draining lymph node on the direct lymphatic pathway from the primary tumor site'. Growing experience with lymphoscintigraphy (LSG) and intraoperative lymphatic mapping makes it clear that there are a myriad anatomic variations of sentinel nodes. Thompson and Uren[2] have suggested a slight modification of Morton's definition: 'any lymph node that receives lymphatic drainage directly from the primary tumor'. This definition helps account for situations in which the primary tumor drains to more than one lymphatic basin, or two lymph nodes in the same lymphatic basin have direct lymphatic communication with the primary tumor (regardless of which appeared first on the lymphoscintigram). A practical problem is how to determine whether two blue-stained or radioactive nodes in a single lymphatic basin are both sentinel nodes, or one is the true sentinel node and the other is a second-echelon node. A second-echelon node receives its lymphatic drainage from the sentinel node, not the primary tumor. The intensity of blue staining cannot be quantified, so if the blue dye looks more intense in one node than in another, what, if anything, does that mean? The radioactivity in nodes can be measured; however, Essner and Morton have described 10 different definitions for a sentinel node based on radioactivity.[3] By any of these definitions, both a sentinel node and a second-echelon node might qualify as sentinel.

From a clinical perspective, what matters? As long as the true sentinel node is removed and analyzed appropriately, it probably does not matter whether a second-echelon node is also removed and treated the same way. When the surgeon is confronted with two radioactive or blue nodes in the same lymphatic basin, usually there is little option except to declare both of them sentinel nodes.

BLUE DYE

The initial work in the identification of the ideal mapping dye was done in animal models. In order to determine the appropriate model, investigators sought a model where the lymphatic drainage mimicked that of the humans. In contrast to almost all other mammals, in which the lymphatic drainage is to a single large lymph node, only the cat has a lymphatic anatomy similar to the multiple lymph nodes found in lymphatic basins of the neck, axilla, or groin in humans.[4] The cat has three inguinal lymph nodes and therefore seemed ideally suited to examine the hypothesis of site-specific lymphatic drainage. The various dyes assessed as potential lymphatic mapping agents have included methylene blue, isosulfan blue, patent blue-V, cyalume, and flourescein.[5]

Methylene blue was not shown to be ideal because of the fact that, when injected intradermally, it has very poor uptake and diffuses rapidly into the surrounding tissue, causing significant staining of the tissue without staining the sentinel node. Cyalume is a fluorescent dye that allows ready identification of the lymphatic channels, but it is associated with significant background fluorescence because of leakage into the surrounding interstitial tissue spaces. It also requires a dark room for visibility. Fluorescein also migrates to the sentinel node; however, it also diffuses into the surrounding tissue, making it difficult to distinguish the sentinel node from the surrounding lymph nodes. The most useful mapping agents that have been found so far are isosulfan blue and patent blue-V dye. Isosulfan blue (Figure 3.1) has a molecular mass of 563.13 Da and is a 2,5-disulfonic acid isomer of patent blue. Approximately 50% of isosulfan blue is weakly bound to serum proteins. Isosulfan blue is rapidly transported through the lymphatics after intradermal injection and is not associated with diffusion into the surrounding tissue. Isosulfan blue is widely available in North America, and patent blue-V dye is widely available in Europe. Occasional shortages of the supply of isosulfan blue forced some clinicians in North America to use methylene blue, with acceptable clinical results[6] (Figure 3.2).

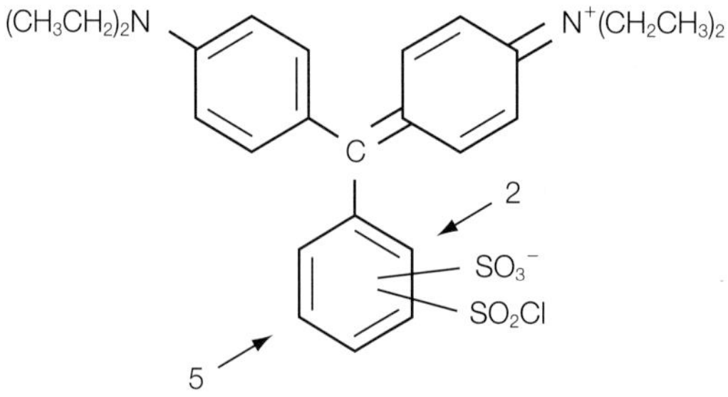

Figure 3.1 Molecular structure of isosulfan blue.

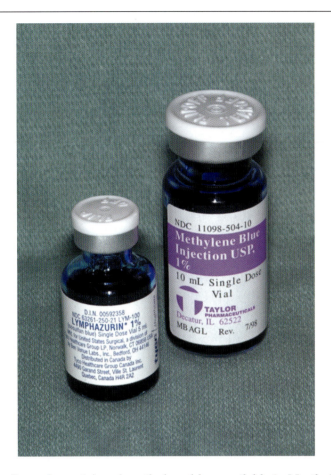

Figure 3.2   Isosulfan blue (Lymphazurin) and methylene blue available in North America.

Technique

Blue dyes are injected into the dermis adjacent to the primary tumor in patients with cutaneous cancers such as melanoma and vulvar cancer. This allows the dye to be taken up into the fine cutaneous lymphatics. Deep subcutaneous injections can result in misleading results when the dye is taken up by deep lymphatics that accompany major blood vessels (see Chapter 1).

The technical approach for sentinel node and lymphatic mapping for vulvar malignancies is as follows. While the patient is under general anesthesia and in the lithotomy position, 2 ml of 1% Lymphazurin (US Surgical Corps, Norwalk, CT, USA) (isosulfan blue) is injected into the dermis at the junction of the tumor and normal tissue. Groin incisions are performed simultaneously in both groins. The surgeon identifies the sentinel node by directly observing the afferent lymphatic channel entering the blue node.

Similarly, in the setting of patients with cervical cancer, after the induction of general anesthesia, while the patient is in the lithotomy position, a laparotomy is performed via a transverse (Maylard or Cherney) or a vertical incision. A sterile speculum is used to expose the cervix for full visualization. A short, 25-gauge needle attached to a needle extender is used to inject 5 ml of Lymphazurin 1% into the mucosa and cervical stroma (5 mm), midway between the cervical os and the rim of the exocervix, in four quadrants. Dargent et al[7] found that injection into the fornix of the vagina led to reduced sentinel node identification. Similarly, O'Boyle found that patients with bulky tumors, where injection into normal cervical mucosa was not possible, also had reduced sentinel node identification rates.[8] The avascular pararectal and paravesical spaces are then developed, with care taken not to disrupt the vascular or lymphatic channels in the nodal basin.

Burke et al[9] described a pilot study for sentinel node identification, using blue dye in patients with endometrial cancer. One-milliliter volumes of isosulfan blue dye 1% are injected into the subserosal myometrium at three midline sites with a tuberculin syringe. Injection sites are the most superior portion of the fundus, the anterior midline being 2 cm below the superior injection site, and the posterior midline 2 cm below the superior injection site. These injection sites are selected to mimic the location of deeply penetrating endometrial tumors arising in any part of the fundus. The injections are performed in the midline to maximize the chances of observing bilateral lymphatic drainage. The retroperitoneal spaces are then opened to expose the aorta, vena cava, and pelvic vessels. Blue lymphatic channels are dissected in an effort to identify dye-containing lymph nodes in these regions.

Safety

As we gain more experience with the use of blue dyes in the identification of sentinel nodes in lymphatic mapping for the various disease sites in gynecologic malignancies, we must remain attentive to the critical factors of safety and the complications of the procedure. One issue of concern with lymphatic mapping is the possibility of iatrogenic tumor spread by injection around and into the tumor. Thus far, to our knowledge, there have been no reports of this event in the literature.

A more concerning event related to the use of blue dyes is the direct side effects caused by these agents. Isosulfan blue is a rosaniline dye of the triphenylmethane type and is the only dye of this type approved for visualization of lymphatics by the Food and Drug Administration in the USA. Evidence suggests that approximately 50% of isosulfan blue, in aqueous solution, is weakly bound to serum proteins, leading to its affinity for lymphatic channels. The primary excretion of isosulfan blue is biliary (90%), and thus patients with hepatobiliary insufficiency may be at an increased risk of complications.[10] The overall complication rate should not exceed 1.5% (package insert).

Urticaria following administration of blue dyes was first reported by Collard and Collette in 1967.[11] Urticaria is an immediate, type I hypersensitivity reaction that is immunoglobulin (Ig) E-dependent. The antigen from isosulfan blue reacts with preformed IgE on the surface of dermal mast cells, causing degranulation. Vasoactive mediators, such as histamine, leukotrienes, and prostaglandins, are released and act on cutaneous venules to cause endothelial cell retraction and gap formation. This increased vascular permeability allows fluid and protein to leak into the superficial dermis, causing urticarial edema.[12] Allergic reactions with localized swelling at the site of administration and mild pruritis of the hands, abdomen, and neck have been described. The mechanism underlying the reaction to isosulfan blue has not been completely elucidated. A massive and direct release of histamine from mast cells and basophils or the activation of the alternative complement pathways has been suggested in prior studies.[13,14] Immunologically, IgE-mediated reactions require a history of previous exposure to compounds of the triphenylmethane family. Prior exposure to these agents may have gone unnoticed, since patent blue and related triphenylmethane dyes are commonly used as antibacterial and antifungal agents and also in several industries such as textiles, paper, and cosmetics.[13]

Anaphylaxis during anesthesia is often a clinical diagnosis presenting, in decreasing frequency, with cardiovascular collapse, erythema, angioedema, bronchospasm (severe or transient), urticaria and/or rash, gastrointestinal symptoms, and pulmonary edema.[15] It is important to understand that during anesthesia, anaphylaxis develops 90% of the time within 10 min after intravenous administration of the causal agent.[16] However, there may be a time delay of 15–30 min observed in cases of anaphylactic reaction to blue dyes, reflecting the fact that these agents are being administered intradermally, rather than intravenously. Once the patient suffers such anaphylactic reaction, the treatment strategy should proceed as follows. The patient should be treated with 100% oxygen, and the intravenous fluid should be increased. Often, more than 5–6 liters of crystalloid may be required, necessitating adequate intravenous access. Persistent tachycardia and low systemic vascular resistance should be treated with 0.2–0.4 mg of intravenous epinephrine. A 5–10-μg/min epinephrine infusion may be needed to maintain hemodynamic stability. Intravenous antihistamines (H1 and H2 blockers) to alter permeability and systemic hemodynamics should be considered if the reaction persists.[17–19] Adverse reactions to isosulfan blue have been confirmed as a rare event. In a series of 406 patients undergoing lymphatic mapping for primary melanoma, Leong et al[17] reported only three cases (1%) of anaphylaxis after intradermal injection of isosulfan blue.

Another systemic manifestation seen after intradermal injections of isosulfan blue is an acute transient or a more prolonged decline in oxygen saturation as measured by pulse oximetry. Coleman et al give a detailed review on the etiology of this phenomenon.[20] Pulse oximetry is a noninvasive modality providing continuous estimations of peripheral tissue oxygen saturation. It functions via determination of the concentrations of oxyhemoglobin and reduced hemoglobin species by measuring the absorbance of light at two wavelengths, 660 and 940 nm, respectively. Isosulfan blue has an absorbance peak of 646 nm (Figure 3.3). In an experiment by Barker et al, the investigators exposed dogs to carbon monoxide over a 3–4-h interval.[21] At a carboxyhemoglobin level of 70%, the Sp_{O_2} values were roughly 90% while the actual Sa_{O_2} was 30%. The pulse oximeter in this case was unable to determine the contribution of carboxyhemoglobin saturation to total saturation; therefore, it grossly overestimated the oxyhemoglobin saturation. Therefore, it is suggested that if the dyes cause abnormal hemoglobin species, they can also influence pulse oximetry measurements.

Another study by Scheller et al confirmed this speculation.[22] These authors showed that injection of 5 ml of intravenous methylene blue could cause large, rapid decreases in Sp_{O_2} without decreases in the actual Sa_{O_2}. In this study, the falsely lowered Sp_{O_2} values were

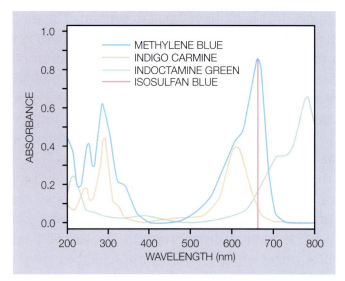

Figure 3.3 Intravenous absorbance spectrum of vital dyes. Note that the absorbance spectrum for isosulfan blue is 646 nm, almost identical to that of oxyhemaglobin. (From Coleman and Whitten[20]).

attributed to absorbance interference at the 660-nm site where oxyhemoglobin is measured. The measurement of oxyhemoglobin is reduced due to competition at this wavelength, and the total calculated saturation (Sp_{O_2}) is reduced. Fortunately, this phenomenon is transient and typically lasts 3–5 min. The inaccuracy of the pulse oximeter in this setting has been confirmed by obtaining arterial blood sampling during the acute fall in Sp_{O_2}, a finding which confirmed adequate and reassuring oxygen saturation. As lymphatic mapping becomes increasingly popular, this effect should be recognized by surgeons and anesthesiologists involved in such cases.

COLLOIDS AND LYMPHOSCINTIGRAPHY (LSG)

The blue staining of a sentinel node with identification of at least one blue-stained afferent lymphatic channel entering the node remains the reference standard for assessment of whether a lymph node is a true sentinel node. However, the introduction of techniques such as radioactive colloid injections and LSG has enhanced the accuracy of detecting the sentinel node. The integral tools when using this approach are a radioactive colloid, a hand-held gamma probe and control box, and a nuclear imaging modality known as a lymphoscintigram.

The primary advantage of using radiocolloid and LSG is that one may detect lymph nodes outside the routine anatomic landmarks of dissection and thus reduce the failure rate of sentinel node identification. In addition, through the use of the gamma probe, the surgeon may specifically target certain areas signaling the presence of a sentinel node that might have been missed by poor uptake of the blue dye and were not detected by the lymphoscintigram.

The ideal radiocolloid must gain access to the lumen of the initial lymphatic channel in sufficient quantity for the lymph vessels to be seen on the dynamic scans. It should combine a rapid and predictable transport toward the sentinel node with persistent retention. The particle size of the radiocolloid is a critical factor in the ease with which these tracers enter the lymphatic system. Large particles (500–2000 nm) remain trapped at the injection site; small particles (4–5 nm) penetrate the capillary membranes and are not available to migrate through the lymphatic channels.[23,24]

In Australia, the most commonly used product is technetium-99m (^{99m}Tc) antimony trisulfide. In Europe, albumin-based compounds are in common use. In North America, the most commonly used radiopharmaceutical is filtered ^{99m}Tc sulfur colloid (^{99m}Tc-SC).[25] This agent has a small particle size (<100 nm), is uniformly dispersed, is highly stable, and, given that it is a gamma emitter, has a short half-life (Table 3.1).

Particles up to 1–2 nm in diameter tend to enter the venous blood system directly. Particles 5–25 nm in size enter lymphatic capillaries via the gaps between cell junctions and the intracellular clefts formed by overlapping cells, which measure 10–25 nm across. Particles up to 75 nm in diameter may gain entry into the lymphatic lumen by pinocytosis.[26] Particles greater than 75 nm in diameter find the connective-tissue lattice increasingly difficult to penetrate, causing most of the injected tracer to remain at the injection site. The first Tc-labeled radiocolloid used for lymphoscintigraphy was unfiltered ^{99m}Tc sulfur colloid, with a range of particle size of 50–2000 nm and an average size of 300 nm. Due to its poor clearance from the injection site, another tracer was needed with smaller particle size; therefore, filtered ^{99m}Tc colloids were developed. This particular agent gains ready access to the lymphatic vessels and migrates rapidly through the vessels to the draining node field, while achieving excellent retention in the lymph nodes for up to 24 hours.[26]

The rate of flow of the injected radiocolloid is also extremely important in the success of sentinel node identification. Once the particles enter the lumen of the lymphatic capillaries, they will move freely and uniformly towards the draining lymph nodes. The valves in the lymphatic vessels will generally not allow any retrograde flow of lymph fluid. It has been previously shown that the movement of tracers along lymphatic capillaries in the skin is very fast.[27] The rate of flow of ^{99m}Tc human serum albumin (HAS) after intradermal injection was found to be 10.4 ± 7.3 cm/min. The average flow rate of ^{99m}Tc antimony sulfur colloid through the lymphatic capillaries following intradermal injection in patients with

Table 3.1 Comparison of radiopharmaceuticals for lymphatic mapping.

	^{99m}Tc-SC	^{99m}Tc-CA	^{99m}Tc-ATL	^{99m}Tc-HAS
Particle size	100–400 nm	5–80 nm	3–30 nm	2–3 nm
Median transit time to SLN	11 min	10 min	n/a	5 min
Dose at injection site at 3 h	76%		83%	
Half-time washout	14 h	8 h		4.3 h

SC: sulfur colloid; CA: colloidal albumin; ATL: antimony trisulfide colloid; HAS: human serum albumin.
(Adapted from Wilhelm et al 1999)

primary cutaneous melanoma was 4.4 cm/min.[28] There is previous evidence that the most important factor affecting flow is the site of intradermal injection of the tracer. The fastest average flow rates were 10 cm/min in the leg and foot, 5.5 cm/min in the forearm and hand, and 4.2 cm/min in the thigh. The slowest average flow rates have been documented in the head and neck (1.5 cm/min).[26] To our knowledge, there is no information in the literature of similar studies in gynecologic malignancies.

Once the injection has been performed, a lymphoscintigram should be performed to visualize the sentinel nodes. In 1953, Sherman and Ter-Pogossian were the first to describe the new technique LSG.[29] This technique allowed the physiology of lymph flow in individual patients to be accurately studied following interstitial injection of a radiocolloid. LSG is a safe, reproducible, and noninvasive technique utilizing radionuclides to image regional lymph node drainage systems. For cutaneous LSG, 10 frames at 1 min per frame is considered adequate to allow the rate of lymph flow to be measured in cm/min. The early dynamic study allows confident identification of sentinel nodes as lymphatic channels drain directly to them.[26] Dynamic images are usually acquired for a total of 20 min. The lymphatic channels are best appreciated by summing the individual dynamic frames to produce a composite dynamic image. Delayed scans are then performed at 2.5–3 h following injection of the radiocolloid tracer. These delayed scans should include all node fields that can possibly receive drainage from the injection site. Each static acquisition should be 5–10 min in length to ensure that even very faint sentinel nodes are detected.[26]

LSG demonstrates a variety of anatomic variations in the number and location of sentinel nodes. Delayed scanning will frequently show more nodal uptake than initial scans. The significance of these additional nodes is not always clear. The most common explanation is that the later-appearing lymph nodes are 'second-echelon nodes', and not sentinel nodes. It is also possible that the additional nodes are also sentinel but with delayed uptake of the radiocolloid due to anatomic factors or local conditions (Figures 3.4 and 3.5).

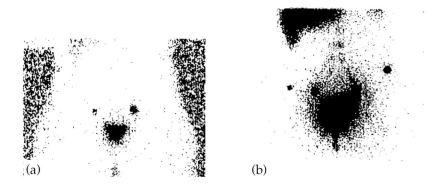

(a) (b)

Figure 3.4 Anterior view of the pelvis 15 min (a) and 1 h (b) following injection of filtered ^{99m}Tc-SC into the cervix. The first image shows bilateral pelvic sentinel nodes. The second image shows what appears to be common iliac and low para-aortic nodes, particularly on the left. These are most likely second-echelon nodes; however, there are lymphatic channels to the common and iliac and aortic nodes directly from the cervix via the posterior lymphatic trunks.

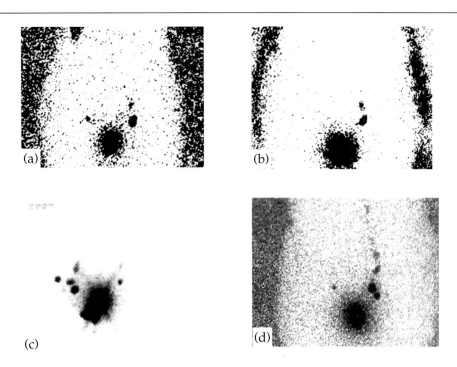

Figure 3.5 Patients with vulvar cancer may have bilateral (a) or unilateral (b) inguinal sentinel nodes depending on the location of the primary tumor. The primary tumor in the patient shown in panel (c) is primarily on the right. These are multiple right inguinal sentinel lymph nodes and one on the left. The patient shown in panel (d) has a tumor primarily on the left. Drainage to second-echelon nodes in the pelvis, and common iliac and low para-aortic nodes are visible, in addition to two inguinal sentinel nodes on delayed images.

The intraoperative detection of the sentinel node relies not only on the visual inspection of the lymphatic basin to identify the 'blue node', but also on the assessment of the radioactive colloid in the sentinel node, or 'hot node', through the aid of a gamma detection device. A gamma detector for surgical use consists of two main components: a hand-held sensor, which contains the gamma-sensitive crystal with a preamplifier, and a reading unit. The efficiency of the detector in the probe is the ratio between the number of gamma photons entering the probe and the number of detected photons. This depends on the crystal material used, on the dimensions (area and thickness) of the crystal, and on the gamma energy.[30] There are two types of detectors: the scintillation detector and the semiconductor detector. The factor that sets them apart is the type of crystal used. The most commonly used detectors are the semiconductor probes, which use a cadmium-telluride or sinc-doped crystal. The advantage of the semiconductor detector is that it generally has a better energy resolution, defined as the ability to discriminate between gamma photons with different energies. In summary, the performance of a gamma detection probe can best be described by the following physical characteristics: sensitivity, spatial (or angular) resolution (collimation), shielding, and energy resolution.[30]

Radioactive decay is a random process; therefore, random fluctuations occur in the measured counts or count rates arising from the decay of radioactivity. When an intraoperative probe is used repeatedly, it will measure the counts or count rates from a given activity of a radiopharmaceutical in a lymph node or tumor. In this setting, a different value is obtained for each measurement. These random fluctuations render the process of measurement of radioactivity an inaccurate one. Sensitivity may be increased by widening the energy window and/or by reducing collimation and shielding. Intraoperative probes are intended for directional counting and must have adequate shielding on the back and sides. Where more precise spatial localization of activity is required, collimation of the detector may be required. Collimation is an extension of the shielding in the forward direction. By lengthening the collimator and/or narrowing its aperture, the detector's field of view is increasingly restricted, additional scatter is excluded, and spatial resolution and detector contrast are improved.[31] In a recent publication by Tiourina et al,[32] the authors provide an extensive review of the main characteristics of a number of probes available for sentinel lymph node detection.

Most intraoperative units consist of a box that plugs into an electrical source and a wand with a cable that plugs into the box. The wand and cable can be placed into a sterile sleeve, so it can be introduced into the operative field while the box is not sterile and off the field. This means that the circulator has to operate the box. A new generation of devices that are battery-operated, compact, and cordless are becoming available that will allow the surgeon to operate alone.

There are a number of other important factors that the surgeon should take into consideration when choosing a gamma detection system. Factors such as the weight and shape of the probe, the visual display and ease of operation, the sound, the hygienic aspects, and, most importantly, the safety are crucial in the process of equipment selection.[30] The weight of the probe is usually determined by the shielding and the collimation; therefore, a thin, light probe may have a small detector area compromising the sensitivity. The shape of the probe is dictated by personal preference. An angle-tip probe may be versatile in that it can be easily manipulated into deep wounds. However, a straight probe has the advantage that the sense of direction is better.[30]

Technique

^{99m}Tc sulfur colloid is injected circumferentially and intradermally at four locations around a cutaneous tumor in patients with melanoma or vulvar cancer the day before surgery. Images are obtained with a gamma camera with a low-energy, high-resolution collimator. Dynamic imaging is performed with 30-s frames for 30 min. An anterior and lateral static image is obtained after 2.5 h. On the day of surgery, an injection of radiocolloid is repeated, before the patient enters the operation room, if more than 18 h have transpired since the patient received the initial injection. Eighteen hours can equal up to three half-lives; therefore, the amount of radiation in the sentinel node will be markedly reduced, making identification more difficult. The lymphoscintigram is brought to the operating room to aid in visualization. The blue dye injection is then performed as described above. Once the groin lymphatic basin has been exposed, the surgeon will perform a quantitative measure of radioactivity in the sentinel node with the gamma probe. The sentinel node is excised separately and measurements are again repeated ex vivo. The lymphatic basin is once again evaluated, visually and with the gamma probe, to identify additional sentinel nodes, and complete lymphadenectomy is then performed. There are various definitions of the sentinel node based on the amount of radioactivity in the node compared with background counts both in vivo and ex vivo; however, there is no universally accepted definition.

In patients with cervical cancer, on the day prior to surgery, the patient's cervix is injected with ^{99m}Tc sulfur colloid in each quadrant around the tumor. Immediately after the injection, dynamic LSG is performed with a gamma camera. The next morning, prior to the surgery, static images are taken, and the patient is brought to the operating room. After the induction of general anesthesia, while the patient is in the lithotomy position, the cervix will be reinvested with ^{99m}Tc sulfur colloid in the same locations as described previously. A laparotomy is then performed via a transverse (Maylard or Cherney) or a vertical incision. The blue dye will be injected. Similarly, the avascular pararectal and paravesical spaces are then developed, with care taken not to disrupt the vascular or lymphatic basins. Hot nodes are identified through the use of a hand-held collimated gamma probe. Once the sentinel node is identified, records are maintained on the anatomic location. The node is subsequently excised separately and sent to pathology for evaluation. The pelvis is re-examined with the hand-held gamma probe to ensure that no other hot nodes remain, and once this is confirmed, the lymphadenectomy is completed.

Safety

There are two areas of concern regarding radiation injury when using radiocolloid: the direct impact on the patient and the effects on the surgical team. Radiation protection is based on three principles, which have been described by the International Commission on Radiological Protection.[33] These include the following: justification—the application of radiation is justified only when the benefit to the exposed individual outweighs the negative consequences; optimization—ensure that the radiation dose to the patient and the general public is 'as low as reasonably achievable'; limitation—boundaries should be placed on risks to individuals to ensure that the risks do not exceed values considered to be acceptable.

The determinant of the radiation dose to which the patient is exposed is the degree of clearance from the site of injection and the lymph node. The clearance of radiocolloids from the interstitial space is very slow; therefore, the largest dose of radiation is delivered to the site of injection. A lesser dose is then received by the lymph nodes, and, subsequently, an even smaller dose is received by the reticuloendothelial system, which will ultimately trap the colloid particles after they have reached the bloodstream.[26] Glass et al[34] evaluated the intralymphatic kinetics of three LSG agents in patients with cutaneous melanoma. The radiopharmaceuticals studied were ^{99}Tc albumin colloid, ^{99}Tc human serum albumin, and

[99]Tc sulfur colloid. They found that ^{99}Tc human serum albumin demonstrated faster washout rates from injections sites and better definition of lymph channels than either particulate agent, whereas particulate agents were retained longer in nodes and demonstrated more nodes in delayed images than in early images. The half-times from the injection site averaged 7.5 ± 6.4 h (^{99}Tc albumin colloid), 4.3 ± 1.4 h (^{99}Tc-HAS), and 13.9 ± 12.7 h (^{99}Tc sulfur colloid). In the event of no migration of the injection radiocolloid after intradermal administration, the maximum absorbed dose using 5 MBq of ^{99}Tc antimony sulfur colloid would be in the order of 0.45 Gy, assuming a volume of distribution of 1 ml. This is considered below the threshold dose for deterministic radiation effects and therefore no erythema or other effect should be seen.[26]

In the USA, the natural background radiation exposes each person to approximately 300 m SI units per year. The annual occupational limits for a radiation worker is a 5-SI units effective dose to the body, 15 SI units to the eye, or 50 SI units to the skin or an individual organ.[35] The distance from the patient to the personnel has a strong effect on the absorbed radiation dose. According to the inverse square law, exposure to radiation diminishes with the square of the distance. In a previous study by Hiller et al,[36] the investigators showed that the doses per case to the surgeon's body and finger with 500 μm ^{99m}Tc were 0.29 and 6.6 m SI units, respectively. The radiation dose to the pathologist will also be low compared with that of the surgeon because of only brief contact with the specimen. The dose to the pathologist's body was 0.052 m SI units.

Based on the concept previously described as optimization, it is generally not recommended for pregnant personnel to perform lymphatic mapping, given that one should always aim for the radiation dose to be 'as low as reasonably achievable'. However, lymphatic mapping should not be a reason to exclude staff from being present in the operating room where the procedure is being performed. The distance to maintain for a pregnant staff member should be at least 1 m from the patient.[37] It is recommended that before introducing the sentinel node procedure, all personnel should be informed about proper handling of material and safety procedures. It is also imperative to monitor radioactive exposure in the hospital setting and have radiation safety monitoring.

EFFICACY

A number of factors may contribute to the failure of sentinel node identification and lymphatic mapping. Partial or complete blockage of the lymphatic channels by metastatic disease will decrease the flow of blue dye and radiocolloid through the system and may decrease the number of nodes visualized on delayed scans. This may also induce collateral lymph flow through other vessels that do not normally drain the primary tumor site. Prior lymphatic or lymph node surgery, as well as prior radiotherapy or trauma to the lymphatic basin, may also lead to alterations in the pattern of lymphatic drainage. This may be associated with a decrease in the number of lymph channels and lymph nodes seen. In addition, the impact of injection of blue dye or radiocolloid to lesions that have been previously partially excised remains to be determined. This may also reflect aberrant lymphatic drainage with subsequent decrease in detection rate. It is also recommended that the sulfur colloid must be fresh and used less than 2 h after preparation, because over time there may be clumping of the colloidal particles, which, in effect, causes them to be larger in size and less effective. Finally, a distinctly important factor that affects on the success rate of sentinel node identification is the technique and expertise of the operating surgeon. Like any other novel technique, lymphatic mapping requires the development of certain skills for which there is a notable learning curve.

Despite the influence of many of the factors discussed above, the majority of the studies published dealing with sentinel node identification and lymphatic mapping in gynecologic malignancies are consistent in the reported detection rates. In vulvar malignancies, Levenback et al[38] were the first to report on the feasibility of intraoperative lymphatic mapping in patients with vulvar cancer. They identified a sentinel node in the groins of 7 of 12 patients (58%), and noted that in each patient in whom the sentinel node was identified, the node correctly reflected the status of the lymphatic basin. In subsequent work, the same group[39] reported on a larger group of patients. A modification from their prior study was an increase in the amount of dye injected into the junction of the tumor. They also changed the time to groin incision from injection from 1 to 5 min and were able to identify the sentinel node in 86% of the patients.

The introduction of LSG for the identification of the sentinel lymph nodes in vulvar cancer was initially reported by DeCesare et al.[40] Intraoperative LSG correctly identified the nodal status as positive in all four cases of metastatic disease and negative in all 16 groins negative for metastasis. In order to attain a large patient accrual, the Gynecologic Oncology Group (GOG) is currently enrolling patients in a study to determine the negative predictive value of sentinel node identification and to evaluate the location of sentinel nodes.

One of the initial attempts of lymphatic mapping for cervical cancer was reported by Echt et al.[41] They described a success rate of 15.4% in identifying the sentinel node. Subsequent work by Verheijen et al[42] revealed findings using LSG, a hand-held gamma probe, and patent blue dye 2.5% (0.2 ml). They reported that LSG showed focal uptake in 6 of 10 eligible patients (60%), the gamma probe identified 8 of 10 patients (80%), and blue staining was seen in only 4 of 10 cases (40%). They concluded that detection by radionuclide results in a higher yield of sentinel node than dye. More recently, Levenback et al[43] showed that preoperative LSG and intraoperative lymphatic mapping are highly successful at identifying sentinel nodes in patients undergoing radical hysterectomy; 100% of patients had at least one sentinel node identified by at least one of the methods. A protocol has been currently approved by the Gynecologic Oncology Group to validate the preliminary results of this technique in cervical cancer by incorporating patients to a multi-institutional trial.

BLUE DYE, RADIOLOCALIZATION, OR BOTH?

Clinicians beginning to perform lymphatic mapping might wonder, 'Should I use one technique or a combination?' The overwhelming consensus in the literature is that a combination of techniques will increase sentinel node identification rates in beginners. In addition, there are clearly clinical situations in which the tumor location is associated with lymphatic drainage to more than one lymphatic basin, and therefore preoperative LSG is mandatory. Examples include head and neck tumors and trunkal melanoma. However, there are clinical situations, such as extremity melanoma, in which LSG does not add much to blue dye, since the lymphatic drainage of the tumor is highly predictable.

Another factor is the availability of the technology involved. In North America, Western Europe, and Australia, funding for cancer research and the ability to obtain new technology and maintain it are high. In other areas of the world, other health-care priorities and budget restraints might prevent acquisition of new technology for cancer. Individual clinicians should be aware of what is available to them and learn to use what is available as well as possible.

CONCLUSION

As we gain additional information in support of the utility of lymphatic mapping and sentinel node in gynecologic malignancies, we strive to pursue this approach so that patient morbidity will be decreased. The potential benefits of sentinel node identification are not limited only to those patients with a positive node. In addition, it may prevent those patients with negative nodes from being exposed to unnecessary additional therapy. Including this procedure in our armamentarium will provide patients with less extensive procedures that not only add important information about prognostic factors but also do not compromise the effectiveness of the surgical intervention. Newer modalities of identifying the sentinel nodes are needed in order to decrease the failure of detection and thus the likelihood of recurrence.

REFERENCES

1. Morton DL, Wen DR, Wong JH, et al. Technical details of intraoperative lymphatic mapping for early stage melanoma. *Arch Surg* 1992;**127**:392–9.
2. Thompson JF, Uren RF. What is a 'sentinel' lymph node? [editorial]. *Eur J Surg Oncol* 2000;**26**:103–4.
3. Essner R, Morton DL. The blue-dye technique. In: Cody HS, ed, *Sentinel Lymph Node Biopsy* (Martin Dunitz: London, 2002) 91–104.

4. Wong JH. Lymphatic drainage of skin in a sentinel lymph node in a feline model. *Ann Surg* 1991;**214**:637–41.

5. Bostick PJ, Giuliano AE. Vital dyes in sentinel node localization. *Semin Nucl Med* 2000;**30**:18–24.

6. Simmons R, Rosenbaum Smith S, Osborne M. Methylene blue dye as an alternative to isosulfan blue dye for sentinel lymph node localization. *Breast J* 2001;**7**:181–3.

7. Dargent D, Martin X, Mathevet P. Laparoscopic assessment of the sentinel lymph node in early stage cervical cancer. *Gynecol Oncol* 2000;**79**:411–15.

8. O'Boyle J, Coleman RL, Bernstein SG, et al. Intraoperative lymphatic mapping in cervix cancer patients undergoing radical hysterectomy: a pilot study. *Gynecol Oncol* 2000;**79**:238–43.

9. Burke TW, Levenback C, Tornos C, et al. Intraabdominal lymphatic mapping to direct selective pelvic and paraaortic lymphadenectomy in women with high-risk endometrial cancers: results of a pilot study. *Gynecol Oncol* 1996;**62**:169–73.

10. Ramirez PT, Levenback C. Sentinel nodes in gynecologic malignancies. *Curr Opin Oncol* 2001;**13**:403–7.

11. Collard M, Collette JM. [Clinical modalities of allergy to patent blue violet]. *J Belge Radiol* 1967;**50**:407–10.

12. Sadiq TS, Burns WW, Taber DJ, et al. Blue urticaria: a previously unreported adverse event associated with isosulfan blue. *Arch Surg* 2001;**136**:1433–5.

13. Gimenez J, Botella Estrada R, Hernandez D, et al. Anaphylaxis after peritumoral injection of sulphan blue 1% for identification of the sentinel node in lymphatic mapping of the breast. *Eur J Surg Acta Chir* 2001;**167**:921–3.

14. Longnecker SM, Guzzardo MM, Van Voris LP. Life-threatening anaphylaxis following subcutaneous administration of isosulfan blue 1%. *Clin Pharm* **4**:219–21.

15. Fisher M, Baldo BA. Anaphylaxis during anaesthesia: current aspects of diagnosis and prevention. *Eur J Anaesthesiol* 1994;**11**:263–84.

16. Moss J. Adverse drug reactions caused by histamine. *Refresh Courses Anesthesiol* 1992;**20**:155–68.

17. Leong SP, Donegan E, Heffernon W, et al. Adverse reactions to isosulfan blue during selective sentinel lymph node dissection in melanoma. *Ann Surg Oncol* 2000;**7**:361–6.

18. Bochner BS, Lichtenstein LM. Anaphylaxis. *N Engl J Med* 1991;**324**:1785–90.

19. Wyatt R. Anaphylaxis. How to recognize, treat and prevent potentially fatal attacks. *Postgrad Med* 1996;**100**:87–90, 96–9.

20. Coleman R, Whitten CW, O'Boyle J, et al. Unexplained decrease in measured oxygen saturation by pulse oximetry following injection of Lymphazurin 1% (isosulfan blue) during a lymphatic mapping procedure. *J Surg Oncol* 1999;**70**:126–9.

21. Barker SJ, Tremper KK. The effect of carbon monoxide inhalation on pulse oximetry and transcutaneous P_{O_2}. *Anesthesiology* 1987;**66**:677–9.

22. Scheller MS, Unger RJ, Kelner MJ. Effects of intravenously administered dyes on pulse oximetry readings. *Anesthesiology* 1986;**65**:550–2.

23. Ege GN. Internal mammary lymphoscintigraphy. The rationale, technique, interpretation and clinical application: a review based on 848 cases. *Radiology* 1976;**118**:101–7.

24. Henze E, Schelbert HR, Collins JD, et al. Lymphoscintigraphy with Tc-99m-labeled dextran. *J Nucl Med* 1982;**23**:923–9.

25. Eshima D, Fauconnier T, Eshima L, et al. Radiopharmaceuticals for lymphoscintigraphy: including dosimetry and radiation considerations. *Semin Nucl Med* 2000;**30**:25–32.

26. Uren RF. The role of nuclear medicine. In: Hiram I, Cody S, eds, *Sentinel Lymph Node Biopsy* (Martin Dunitz: London, 2002) 19–43.

27. Nathanson SD, Nelson L, Karvelis KC. Rates of flow of technetium 99m-labeled human serum albumin from peripheral injection sites to sentinel lymph nodes. *Ann Surg Oncol* 1996;**3**:329–35.

28. Uren RF, Howman Giles RB, Thompson JF, et al. Variability of cutaneous lymphatic flow rates in melanoma patients. *Melanoma Res* 1998;**8**:279–82.

29. Sherman A, Ter-Pogossian M. Lymph-node concentration of radioactive colloidal gold following interstitial injection. *Cancer* 1953;**6**:1238–40.

30. Muller S, Sazonova-Tiourina T, Jan Arends A. Comparison of the physical characteristics of different gamma detection devices. In: Nieweg OE, et al, eds, *Lymphatic Mapping and Probe Applications in Oncology* (Marcel Dekker: New York, 2000) 87–100.

31. Zanzonico P, Heller S. The intraoperative gamma probe: basic principles and choices available. *Semin Nucl Med* 2000;**30**:33–48.

32. Tiourina T, Arends B, Huysmans D, et al. Evaluation of surgical gamma probes for radioguided sentinel node localisation. *Eur J Nucl Med* 1998;**25**:1224–31.

33. 1990 Recommendations of the International Commission on Radiological Protection. *Ann ICRP* 1991;**21**:1–201.

34. Glass EC, Essner R, Morton DL. Kinetics of three lymphoscintigraphic agents in patients with cutaneous melanoma. *J Nucl Med* 1998;**39**:1185–90.

35. Fiorica JV, Grendys E, Hoffman M. Intraoperative radiolocalization of the sentinel node in patients with vulvar cancer. *Operative Tech Gynecol Surg* 2001;**6**:27–32.

36. Hiller D, Royal H. Intraoperative gamma radiation detection and radiation safety. In: Whitman E, Reintgen D, eds, *Radioguided Surgery* (Landes Bioscience: Austin, TX, 1999) 23–38.

37. Pijpers R, Meijer S, Dignum PH, et al. Radiation protection in the sentinel procedure. In: Nieweg OE, et al, eds, *Lymphatic Mapping and Probe Applications in Oncology* (Marcel Dekker: New York, 2000) 213–24.

38. Levenback C, Burke TW, Gershenson DM, et al. Intraoperative lymphatic mapping for vulvar cancer. *Obstet Gynecol* 1994;**84**:163–7.

39. Levenback C, Burke TW, Morris M, et al. Potential applications of intraoperative lymphatic mapping in vulvar cancer. *Gynecol Oncol* 1995;**59**:216–20.

40. DeCesare SL, Fiorica JV, Roberts WS, et al. A pilot study utilizing intraoperative lymphoscintigraphy for identification of the sentinel lymph nodes in vulvar cancer. *Gynecol Oncol* 1997;**66**:425–8.

41. Echt M, Finan MA, Hoffman MS, et al. Detection of sentinel lymph nodes with lymp-hazurin in cervical, uterine, and vulvar malignancies. *South Med J* 1999;**92**:204–8.

42. Verheijen R, Pijpers R, Van Diest PJ, et al. Sentinel node detection in cervical cancer. *Obstet Gynecol* 2000;**96**:135–8.

43. Levenback C, Coleman RL, Burke TW, et al. Lymphatic mapping and sentinel node identification in patients with cervix cancer undergoing radical hysterectomy and pelvic lymphadenectomy. *J Clin Oncol* 2002;**20**:688–93.

4 ULTRASTAGING OF THE SENTINEL NODE

Paul J. van Diest and Ate van der Zee

INTRODUCTION

The main task for the pathologist is to examine sentinel nodes (SNs) for possible metastasis.[1–5] This examination has to be done with more attention ('ultrastaging') than the usual central HE section, since a false-negative SN assessment leading to omission of lymph node dissection may lead to untreatable locoregional tumor outgrowth in tumor-bearing lymph nodes that have been left behind. The SN evaluation will usually be done postoperatively. If indicated, a complete lymph node dissection would then be performed in a second session. However, it would be a great advantage to the patient and surgeon if the regional lymph node dissection, when necessary, could be performed in the same operating session as the SN procedure and the excision of the primary tumor. This requires accurate and efficient intraoperative assessment of the SN by the pathologist. There are several ways for postoperative and intraoperative SN evaluation. These include histopathologic investigation, immunohistochemistry (IHC), imprint cytology, fine-needle aspiration cytology, flow cytometry, and molecular biologic analysis. Several review papers on the pathology of the SN have been published.[1,5,6] The aim of this chapter is to provide an up-to-date discussion of the virtues and flaws of these different methods, and to present practical guidelines for the SN investigation in gynecologic cancers.

INTRAOPERATIVE RAPID ANALYSIS

Frozen section

As just briefly mentioned, it would be a great advantage to the patient and surgeon if the regional lymph node dissection, when necessary, could be performed in the same operating session as the SN procedure and the excision of the primary tumor. This requires accurate and efficient intraoperative assessment of the SN by the pathologist, which can be done by frozen-section analysis. This is usually done by a single HE frozen section. The next paragraphs will make clear that without step sections and IHC, up to 15–20% of metastases may be missed in patients with breast cancer or cutaneous melanoma. Therefore, the theoretical sensitivity for detection of metastases by single HE frozen section analysis is (under optimal conditions) not higher than 80–85%, and lower in more difficult conditions as is often the case with frozen sections.

In an initial study from the VU University Medical Center on 54 breast cancer patients,[7] 27 of 31 SN metastases were detected by the frozen-section procedure. The sensitivity of this frozen-section procedure was 87%, the specificity 100%, the positive predictive value 100%, and the negative predictive value 91%. These data compare very well with some other initial studies.[8–10] However, these initial good results have raised expectations too high with regard to the sensitivity of the SN frozen section. In a larger follow-up study, our sensitivity dropped to about 60% when the percentage of lobular carcinomas had increased, and frozen sections were also routinely analyzed by less experienced pathologists, leading to some judgment errors.[11] These observations have been confirmed by others.[12,16] In general, the ability of the frozen sections to detect metastases is clearly higher for macrometastases than micrometastases.[16]

Although the sensitivity of the single HE frozen section is clearly not optimal, those patients that are positive by this technique can still undergo immediate axillary lymph node dissection, and this is an obvious advantage. However, a significant percentage of frozen-section-negative patients will appear to have micrometastases in the final HE or IHC sections, and in these patients axillary lymph node dissection will have to be considered as a second operation.

Veronesi et al[17] described a combination of intraoperative step frozen sections with rapid IHC to arrive at an intraoperative final diagnosis in breast cancer, correctly predicting a metastasis-free SN in 95.4% of cases.[18] This procedure was, however, very labor-intensive and led to a significant increase in the operating time (up to 1 h). Zurrida et al[19] devised a similar but quicker intraoperative method, requiring about 40 min, in which pairs of sections were taken every 50 μm for the first 15 sections and every 100 μm thereafter, sampling the entire node. This extensive intraoperative frozen examination correctly predicted an uninvolved axilla in 95.3% of cases. Ultraquick IHC protocols are mandatory for this.[20] In another study using extensive intraoperative sampling taking up to 60 sections per SN,[9] HE section analysis by an experienced pathologist proved more important than IHC, and this method had the accuracy of a definitive histologic examination. The frozen-section procedure should not be essentially different for cervical adenocarcinomas and vulvar and cervical squamous cell carcinomas.[21]

In frozen-section analysis, care must be taken that the tissue is frozen flat (as by freezing it with a cooled flat weight on top of it), and that cutting is performed cautiously to prevent inadvertent tissue loss as much as possible. Intraoperative step sections are time-consuming and lead to excessive tissue loss, and extra sections for the different levels need to be cut immediately for IHC.[17] Nevertheless, it is unavoidable that some SN material will be lost; theoretically, this may lead to missing some SN micrometastases. The chance of this occurring will naturally depend on the size and the distribution of the micrometastases. However, since the likelihood of second-echelon lymph nodes containing metastases correlates to the size of the SN metastasis,[22,23] this risk may be acceptable. The percentage of SN metastases discarded during tissue processing is probably quite low when proper measures to prevent tissue loss are taken, since the percentage of SN metastases found in a VU University Medical Center study in breast cancer[7] was comparable to that in all other breast cancer studies without an intraoperative procedure.[24–26] Moreover, it has to be realized that for the average lymph node, only about 1% of the total node volume is actually looked at under the microscope, even when making step sections and performing IHC.

In our view, the disadvantage of potentially missing some micrometastases due to loss of tissue is outweighed by the advantage of performing full lymph node dissection during the initial operation in SN-positive cancer patients and by the increased number of lymph node metastases found by the more detailed investigation of the SN compared to usual locoregional lymph nodes. The operative delay of 15–20 min caused by the frozen-section investigation is acceptable, since during this time the primary tumor can be excised.

Imprint cytology

Imprint slides can simply be produced from lymph nodes by firmly pressing the cut surface to a glass slide. In a postoperative and intraoperative setting, the May-Grünwald-Giemsa and Quickdiff stains, respectively, allow detection of metastatic cells. Imprint cytology has previously been described as helpful in the detection of lymph node metastases of prostate[27] and breast cancer.[28,29] Fisher et al[29] detected breast cancer axillary lymph node metastases intraoperatively in imprints of 18/21 (86%) patients. In an intraoperative study in breast cancer,[7] imprints were prepared from all cut SN surfaces, showing a sensitivity of imprints for detection of SN metastases of 62% with a specificity of 100%. The sensitivity of the imprints was significantly lower than that of frozen sections. In addition, there were no SNs in which the imprints convincingly showed metastases while the frozen sections did not. Therefore, we found that imprints did not have more value than the intraoperative, frozen-section SN investigation.

However, other authors have had much better experience. Motomura et al[30] described a sensitivity of intraoperative imprint cytology of breast cancer SNs of 91%, a result which was better than HE frozen-section analysis. Turner et al[14] used a combination of frozen-section analysis and imprints, resulting in a high sensitivity. Ratanawichitrasin et al[31] observed an imprint sensitivity of 82% compared to HE final sections (no IHC), a result which is comparable to the experience of Cserni.[32] The imprint method therefore seems to be reasonably useful for intraoperative SN evaluation.

Interestingly, the perception of the surgeon of the importance of false-negative and false-positive results appears to be changing. Reasoning from the fact that, traditionally, the complete lymph node dissection is the standard therapy, one could argue that false-positive results are not really a problem, and that false-negative results are practically a bigger problem since a second operation will then be necessary. However, the growing reliability and importance of the SN procedure will soon put more emphasis on the impact of false-positive results, since they would lead to an 'unnecessary' lymph node dissection.

SERIAL SECTIONING

The SNs are fixed in neutral buffered formaldehyde and completely embedded after lamellating them according to their size. Various protocols for lamellating have been advocated. Our preferred way is as follows: SNs smaller than 0.5 cm are processed and paraffin-embedded intact, those between 0.5 and 1 cm are halved, and those larger than 1 cm are lamellated into pieces of approximately 0.5 cm in size (Figure 4.1). It has been suggested that tumor cells preferentially enter the SNs through the contralateral side of the hilum of lymph nodes.[33] If true, this would have important consequences, since bisecting the long axis of the SN from the outer capsule to hilum would produce two cut surfaces of the midline region where the first single tumor cell or small groups of tumor cells would be readily visible. However, experimental evidence for this theory is lacking, and, in practice, it is quite difficult to identify the hilum.

From an average lymph node, several thousand sections can be produced. As this obviously confronts the pathologist with an unacceptably high workload, a compromise has to be found between workload and sensitivity, which will unavoidably lead to missing some tumor cells. This compromise is best achieved by taking step sections at regular intervals, increasing the percentage of metastases found in SNs with about 8%,[34,35] depending on the protocol used (Table 4.1). In vulvar squamous cell cancer,[21,36–39] the yield of step sectioning and IHC seems to be lower. In vulvar cancer, De Hullu et al[36] detected by step sectioning and IHC, in 102 sentinel lymph nodes that were negative on routine examination, four additional metastases (4%; 95% CI, 1–9%). Three of the four metastases were observed in patients whose lymph nodes were negative on routine examination. One additional metastasis was found in a patient who already had another SN with metastatic disease. In squamous cell cervical cancer, Levenback et al[21] detected, in 31 patients with no positive SNs on routine HE processing, no micrometastases with serial step sectioning. Ten patients with negative SNs on routine HE and serial step sectioning had their SNs submitted to cytokeratin IHC analysis. No metastases were identified with this technique. One patient with a

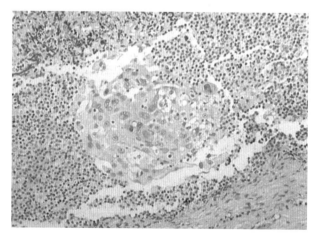

Figure 4.1   Lymph node metastasis at routine histopathologic examination (Hematoxylin and eosin staining, ×200 microscope magnification).

Table 4.1 Cumulative number of patients with breast cancer sentinel node metastases found with each additional level (250-mm intervals) in a total of 86 patients (HE;[hematoxylin/eosin] staining, IHC; CAM5.2 IHC). (Adapted from Torrenga et al.[34])

	HE positive	% HE positive	IHC positive	% IHC positive
Level 1	69	80	74	86
Level 2	71	83	77	90
Level 3	73	85	81	94
Level 4	75	87	84	98
Level 5	76	88	86	100

IHC: immunohistochemistry.

positive SN on routine HE staining had a micrometastasis found by serial sectioning of the contralateral sentinel node.[21]

Step sections are obviously necessary only when the first section appears to be tumor negative. In cutting the step ribbons, one section of each ribbon should be mounted for HE staining, while the rest of the ribbon should be saved for eventual IHC (see below). Although mucin histochemical stains (PAS and Alcian blue) may be useful for detecting adenocarcinoma metastases, especially in primary lobular breast cancer, IHC is a much more sensitive method (see below).

IMMUNOHISTOCHEMISTRY (IHC)

IHC is a generally applicable and cost-effective technique that has proven to be very useful for detection of tumor cells in lymph nodes (especially micrometastases) by demonstration of proteins that are, within the context of the tissue analyzed, tumor specific (Figures 4.2 and 4.3). Overall, IHC increases the percentage of metastases found in non-SN

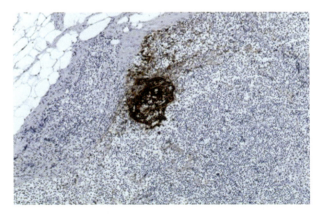

Figure 4.2 Lymph node metastasis confirmed with immunohistopathologic examination (AE1/3 immunohistochemical staining ×100 microscope magnification).

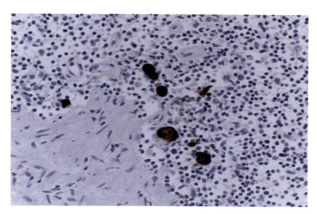

Figure 4.3 Scattered keratin-positive cells in a sentinel lymph node. The clinical significance of this finding in gynecologic cancers is not known (AE1/3 immunohistochemical staining ×400 microscope magnification).

lymph nodes by, on average, 20%,[1] the gain being highest in lobular breast cancer. For the SN, the range of conversion of the SN to positive by ultrastaging (however, with quite varying protocols) is 2–20%, with an average of 11% (Table 4.2).

Different antibodies have been used for breast cancer, of which CAM5.2 seems to be the one most widely used. In general, no background staining is seen with this antibody, and its sensitivity is about 100%. Caveats are epithelial and mesothelial inclusions. Staining of sinus-lining cells may sometimes be observed, especially when using automated immunostainers, but sinus-lining cells are easily recognized morphologically. CAM5.2 is also useful for metastases of adenocarcinomas from most other sites. EMA and other MUC1

Table 4.2 Overview of different studies evaluating the conversion rate of SNs to positive by immunohistochemistry (IHC).

Study	Organ	No. of patients converted to positive by IHC	% Converted
Jannink 1998[68]	Breast	3/19	16
Pendas 1999[69]	Breast	41/385	11
Schreiber 1999[70]	Breast	17/210	9
Kowolik 2000[71]	Breast	2/33	6
Liu 2000[15]	breast	5/38	13
Hsieh 2000[72]	Breast	1/41	2
de Hullu 2000[36]	Vulva	3/23	13
Terada 2000[73]	Vulva	2/14	14
Torrenga 2001[34]	Breast	17/86	20
Mann 2001[74]	Breast	10/51	20
Molpus 2001[75]	Vulva	2/18	11
Levenback[21]	Cervix	0/31	0%
Overall		*103/949*	*11%*

antibodies have too low a specificity, since they may also stain plasma cells and macrophages, and the sensitivity of EMA is also low, since breast cancers and other adenocarcinomas can well be EMA negative. CEA and NCRC11 are specific, but not very sensitive.

For squamous cell carcinomas metastases, AE1/3 is a reliable antibody. It has high specificity and sensitivity. Van den Brekel et al[40] found additional non-SN lymph node metastases in 3/13 head and neck squamous cell carcinoma patients (23%) with this antibody. This antibody can also be used for squamous, gynecologic cancer; however, its yield appears to be modest, as described in the previous paragraph.

FINE-NEEDLE ASPIRATION CYTOLOGY

A few studies have explored the possibility of ultrasonographically guided fine-needle aspiration biopsy (FNAB) to detect SN metastases. Motomura et al[41] examined the axillae of 60 patients with breast cancer, in whom a hot spot was detected by gamma probe, by ultrasonography. Preoperative diagnosis of SN metastasis by gamma probe and ultrasonographically guided FNAB was compared with the histologic results of SN. SNs were visualized by ultrasonography in 29 of 60 patients (48%). The sensitivity, specificity, and overall accuracy of ultrasonography in the diagnosis of SN metastasis were 50%, 92%, and 77%, respectively. Of 14 patients with positive results by ultrasonography, four had positive and two had negative cytology. The combination of ultrasonography and ultrasonographically guided FNAB for visualized nodes had a sensitivity of 79%, specificity of 93%, and overall accuracy of 86%. Blind FNAB in the hot spot was not useful in the detection of SN metastasis in patients whose SNs failed to be detected by ultrasonography. Gamma probe and ultrasonographically guided FNAB is therefore a potentially useful method for preoperative detection of SN metastasis. In patients with positive SN FNAB, further SN biopsy is no longer indicated and complete axillary lymph node dissection can be performed as a primary procedure. There are at present no data on the value of FNAB for vulvar and cervical cancer.

FLOW CYTOMETRY (FCM)

Flow cytometry (FCM) is a technique of measuring properties of cells in suspension after staining with a fluorescent dye. It is a fast technique in which thousands of cells can be screened in minutes. The first FCM approach for detection of metastases in lymph nodes is with the same antibodies as for IHC, coupled with a fluorescent tag. However, such FCM is not very suitable for detecting rare events, so the additional value to extensive histopathology is probably very limited. The second approach is DNA FCM, in which a clone of cells with abnormal DNA content or a high percentage of S-G2M-phase cells may indicate metastatic cells. Joensuu et al[42] found the diagnostic accuracy of such DNA FCM analysis of fine-needle aspirations of lymph nodes to be 92%, with a sensitivity of 91% and a specificity of 95%. DNA FCM suggested the correct diagnosis in five of the seven cytologically false-negative cases and in nine of the 12 cytologically indeterminate or suspicious cases.

A more sophisticated approach is a DNA/cytokeratin double-staining procedure, as described by Leers et al.[43] In this study, the breast cancer paraffin pieces that were left over between step ribbons were used to prepare single-cell suspensions with preservation of the cytoplasm, so that epithelial cells could then be identified by cytokeratin staining. The presence of [CLOSECHEV]1% epithelial cells was very indicative of metastases, but cell cycle parameters of the epithelial fraction (DNA aneuploidy or high percentage of S-phase) provided further evidence. By this approach, metastases were found that were not detected by HE and IHC.

MOLECULAR TECHNIQUES

An even more refined molecular biologic approach to the detection of micrometastases is amplification by reverse-transcriptase polymerase chain reaction (RT-PCR) of mRNA, which is expressed in the cancer cells of interest, but not by other lymph node cells. By dilution experiments,[44,45] it has been estimated that a single cancer cell can be detected by RT-PCR among 10^6–10^7 normal cells. This indicates that RT-PCR is by far the most sensitive method for detection of metastases in SNs.

Different studies have evaluated the usefulness of RT-PCR for detecting SN metastases. Schoenfeld et al[46] compared keratin 19 RT-PCR with histopathologic results (HE and IHC) in axillary lymph nodes of breast cancer patients, and found all 18 histopathologically involved lymph nodes to be positive by RT-PCR. Of the 39 lymph nodes that were histologically negative, 14 were positive by RT-PCR. Noguchi et al[44,47] compared MUC1 and keratin 19 RT-PCR, and found all 10 lymph nodes that were histopathologically positive to be also positive by RT-PCR, and that three (6%) and five (9%) of histopathologically negative (HE only) lymph nodes expressed MUC1 and keratin 19, respectively, indicating the presence of metastases. Hoon et al[45] found occult metastases by β-HCG RT-PCR in 25% of patients that were histopathologically lymph node negative, and Kataoka et al[48] found conversion percentages of 25% for CEA and 21% for mammoglobin in an HE-only study. In this last study, RT-PCR improved the prediction of axillary lymph node status to 98.5%. In a study on breast and gastrointestinal cancer, Mori et al[49] detected metastases by CEA RT-PCR in 47/87 (54%) lymph nodes that were negative on regular histology. Wascher et al,[50] using MAGE-A3 RT-PCR, found 28 of 73 (38%) histopathologically negative SNs to be RT-PCR positive. Manzotti et al[51] found a high prevalence of positive RT-PCR in histologically uninvolved SNs when considering single markers, but when at least two of three markers (maspin, cytokeratin 19, and mammaglobin) were expressed, the concordance with either SN or axillary lymph node status was highest.[51] Some authors[52] use RT-PCR routinely. For vulvar cancer, there are at present no data on the value of RT-PCR . Van Trappen et al[53] applied a fully quantitative, real-time RT-PCR assay to document absolute copy numbers of the epithelial marker cytokeratin 19 in primary tumors, 156 lymph nodes from 32 patients with cervical cancer (stages IA2, IB1, and IB2), and 32 lymph nodes from nine patients with benign disease. All primary tumors and histologically involved lymph nodes (six) had increased expression of cytokeratin 19 mRNA, while lower expression of cytokeratin 19 was detected in 66 (44%) of 150 histologically uninvolved lymph nodes, and in nodes from 16 of 32 patients with cervical cancer. Fifteen of these 16 patients with evidence of micrometastases had the highest cytokeratin 19 transcription level in a first lymph node drainage station. Transcription of cytokeratin 19 was found at a low level in just one of 32 lymph nodes obtained from nine patients with benign disease. The median copy number of cytokeratin 19 transcription was significantly higher in association with adverse prognostic features. These results suggest that about 50% of early-stage cervical cancers shed tumor cells to the pelvic lymph nodes, and the amount of cytokeratin 19 expression was related to clinicopathologic features. However, further studies are required to document the clinical implications of molecular micrometastases.[53]

These studies underline the great promise of RT-PCR for detecting SN metastases. However, several comments have to be made. First, a clear drawback of all of the above studies is that those pieces that were examined had not been subjected to the usual histopathologic investigation with HE and IHC. If this had been done, more metastases might well have been detected with these conventional methods as well. Concluding that the molecular analysis is superior is therefore tricky. A better approach seems to be to subject those pieces to molecular analysis that would normally be thrown away: the pieces between the step sections. However, this requires that RNA be successfully extracted from paraffin-embedded tissue. This appears to be possible, as was shown by Palmieri et al for melanoma,[54] although the sensitivity of paraffin RT-PCR may be lower than that of frozen tissue. Second, contamination is a big potential problem, and histopathologic control of specimens homogenized for blind assays such as RT-PCR will always be necessary. A pitfall is epithelial or mesothelial inclusion. Third, healthy volunteers appear to express presumed specific markers, such as CEA, CK-19, GA733.2, and MUC-1,[55] in their blood and lymph nodes, meaning that these markers can yield false-positive results. Fourth, one must ask whether the high sensitivity of RT-PCR has clinical significance. As shown in several studies, second-echelon breast cancer metastases are hardly ever found when the true SN is negative by extensive histopathologic investigation with step sections and IHC.[26] It remains to be proven that RT-PCR may identify those few patients that escape extensive histopathologic investigation, but, especially for melanoma, there is promise.

However, overall, RT-PCR may be a relatively quick and cheap alternative,[56] so further studies are necessary to develop combinations of primers that are specific enough to establish the role of RT-PCR in detecting metastases in SNs, and to assess the clinical value of RT-PCR. Promising first results have been described.[57]

CONCLUSIONS

The optimal standard protocol?

Unfortunately, there is no consensus among different groups as to how many step sections are needed, and what the step size should be. Recent studies have provided breast cancer SN data that are useful to arrive at evidence-based guidelines in this respect.[26,33–35] Turner et al[33] examined 60 SNs by step HE sections and cytokeratin IHC at 10 levels separated by 40 µm, following the hilum approach. Levels 1 and 2 yielded additional micrometastases in nine SNs (15%), but in levels 3–10, only two (3%) further metastases were found. They therefore recommended the study of only two levels separated by 40 µm. However, their SN slices were 2–3 mm thick, so even with 10 levels at 40 µm, only 400 µm would be investigated, accounting for no more than 13–20% of the SN slices. This seems to be insufficient, and may explain the disappointing yield of this procedure. Rather than taking many sections at small intervals, it may be more efficient to take fewer sections at larger step intervals. In the study of Cserni,[58] SNs were serially sectioned and every 10th–20th level was examined by HE and/or IHC. A central cross-section through the SN would have failed to detect metastases in 8/26 lymph nodes (31%), leading to a false-negative SN status in 6/21 patients (29%). The percentage of metastases found increased from 69% with only a central cross-section to 77% with five further steps, to 81% with 10 steps, and to 96% with 15 steps. Only at 45 steps was a 100% sensitivity found. Cserni stated that with a three-level approach at 25%, 50%, and 75% of the block, metastases would have been missed in 15% of patients. A previous non-SN study by Zhang et al[59] found almost all metastases with such a three-level approach. Our own SN protocol includes step sectioning at five levels with an interval of 250 µm with HE and IHC when the first-level HE section is negative.[1,2,6,7,34,35,60–64] Since we perform frozen-section analysis routinely, leading to some loss of material, this ensures sampling through the better part of the SN. In practice, this has proven to provide an acceptable workload. The yield per level has been detailed, as shown in Table 4.1.[34] When we take the cumulative total of detected metastases at level 5 to be 100%, the percentage of SN-positive patients increased from 80%, 83%, 85%, 87% to 88% in the HE sections through levels 1–5, and with IHC from 86%, 90%, 94%, 98% to 100%. With a similar protocol, an even higher conversion rate was found by Dowlatshahi et al.[65] The clinical relevance of finding micrometastases on the higher levels is underlined by the fact that three of nine patients in whom single-cell metastases were detected only at levels 3–5 had metastases in the subsequent axillary lymph node dissection. Besides, we have seen several breast cancer cases with only a few metastatic cells in the SN detected by IHC, while second-echelon lymph nodes contained significant metastatic deposits.[22,66] This is probably due to rerouting of the lymph drainage because of lymph obstruction of the 'real' SN by the heavy tumor load. Others have also reported relatively high percentages of involved non-SNs in SN micrometastases.[67] IHC is therefore essential when the initial HE SN (step) sections are all negative, and ribbons must be kept when step-cutting.

Table 4.3 Recommendations for the SN evaluation (IHC: immunohistochemistry).

Adenocarcinoma (breast, cervix)	Single HE frozen section analysis and/or imprint cytology. HE step sections (5 with 250-μm interval) with CAM5.2 IHC.
Squamous cell cancer (vulva, cervix)	Single HE frozen-section analysis with imprint cytology. HE step sections (5 with 250-μm interval) with AE1/3 IHC.

Therefore, in our opinion, there is sufficient evidence to recommend this as the current optimal protocol (Table 4.3). Future studies may help to make SN sampling more efficient when the hilum approach is better validated.

Summary remarks

Ultrastaging, including step HE-stained sections and IHC, is mandatory for reliable detection of metastases in SNs of gynecologic cancers. Intraoperative single HE frozen-section and imprint cytologic analysis of SNs has been shown to be reasonably reliable for detection of breast cancer metastases, but a false-negative rate of 30–40% will have to be accepted. These are all standard techniques that are available in each pathology laboratory, so nothing special, except the dedication of the pathologist, is required. Although the workload for a SN is high for the pathologist, it should be borne in mind that there will be fewer axillary lymph node dissection specimens to handle, saving time. Altogether, the SN procedure may save costs.[8] Further studies are necessary to establish the role of FCM and sophisticated molecular biologic techniques such as RT-PCR in detecting SN metastases. Table 4.3 summarizes our current recommendations for the SN evaluation and ultrastaging in different gynecologic cancers.

REFERENCES

1. Van Diest PJ, Peterse HL, Borgstein PJ, et al. Pathologic investigation of sentinel lymph nodes. *Eur J Nuclear Med* 1999;**26**:S43–A9.
2. Van Diest PJ. Histopathologic workup of sentinel lymph nodes: how much is enough? *J Clin Pathol* 1999;**52**:871–3.
3. Cserni G. How to improve low lymph node recovery rates from axillary clearance specimens of breast cancer. A short-term audit. *J Clin Pathol* 1998;**51**:846–9.
4. Cserni G. The reliability of sampling three to six nodes for staging breast cancer. *J Clin Pathol* 1999;**52**:681–3.
5. Cserni G. Axillary staging of breast cancer and the sentinel node. *J Clin Pathol* 2000;**53**:733–41.

6. Van Diest PJ, Torrenga H, Meijer S, et al. Pathologic analysis of sentinel lymph nodes. *Semin Surg Oncol* 2001;**20**:238–45.

7. Van Diest PJ, Torrenga H, Borgstein PJ, et al. Reliability of intra-operative frozen section and imprint cytological investigation of sentinel lymph nodes in breast cancer. *Histopathology* 1999;**35**:14–18.

8. Flett MM, Going JJ, Stanton PD, et al. Sentinel node localization in patients with breast cancer. *Br J Surg* 1998;**85**:991–3.

9. Galimberti V, Zurrida S, Intra M, et al. Sentinel node biopsy interpretation: the Milan experience. *Breast J* 2000;**6**:306–9.

10. Viale G, Bosari S, Mazzarol G, et al. Intraoperative examination of axillary sentinel lymph nodes in breast carcinoma patients. *Cancer* 1999;**85**:2433–8.

11. Rahusen FD, Pijpers R, Van Diest PJ, et al. The implementation of the sentinel node biopsy as a routine procedure for patients with breast cancer. *Surgery* 2000;**128**:6–12.

12. Gulec SA, Su J, O'Leary JP, et al. Clinical utility of frozen section in sentinel node biopsy in breast cancer. *Am Surg* 2001;**67**:529–32.

13. Tanis PJ, Boom RP, Koops HS, et al. Frozen section investigation of the sentinel node in malignant melanoma and breast cancer. *Ann Surg Oncol* 2001;**8**:222–6.

14. Turner RR, Hansen NM, Stern SL, et al. Intraoperative examination of the sentinel lymph node for breast carcinoma staging. *Am J Clin Pathol* 1999;**112**:627–34.

15. Liu LH, Siziopikou KP, Gabram S, et al. Evaluation of axillary sentinel lymph node biopsy by immunohistochemistry and multilevel sectioning in patients with breast carcinoma. *Arch Pathol Lab Med* 2000;**124**:1670–3.

16. Weiser MR, Montgomery LL, Susnik B, et al. Is routine intraoperative frozen-section examination of sentinel lymph nodes in breast cancer worthwhile? *Ann Surg Oncol* 2000;**7**:651–5.

17. Veronesi U, Zurrida S, Galimberti V. Consequences of sentinel lymph node in clinical decision making in breast cancer and prospects for future studies. *Eur J Surg Oncol* 1998;**24**:93–5.

18. Veronesi U, Zurrida S, Mazzarol G, et al. Extensive frozen section examination of axillary sentinel nodes to determine selective axillary dissection. *World J Surg* 2001;**25**:806–8.

19. Zurrida S, Mazzarol G, Galimberti V, et al. The problem of the accuracy of intraoperative examination of axillary sentinel nodes in breast cancer. *Ann Surg Oncol* 2001;**8**:817–20.

20. Richter T, Nährig J, Komminoth P, et al. Protocol for ultra-rapid immunostaining of frozen sections. *J Clin Pathol* 1999;**52**:461–3.

21. Levenback C, Coleman RL, Burke TW, et al. Lymphatic mapping and sentinel node identification in patients with cervix cancer undergoing radical hysterectomy and pelvic lymphadenectomy. *J Clin Oncol* 2002;**20**:688–93.

22. Rahusen FD, Van Diest PJ, Meijer S. Re: Chu et al; do all patients with sentinel node metastasis from breast carcinoma need complete axillary node dissection? *Ann Surg* 2000;**231**:615–6.

23. Chu KU, Turner RR, Hansen NM, et al. Do all patients with sentinel node metastasis from breast carcinoma need complete axillary node dissection? *Ann Surg* 1999;**229**:536–41.

24. Giuliano AE. Sentinel lympadenectomy in primary breast carcinoma: an alternative to routine axillary dissection. *J Surg Oncol* 1996;**62**:75–6.

25. Veronesi U, Paganelli G, Galimberti V, et al. Sentinel-node biopsy to avoid axillary dissection in breast cancer with clinically negative lymph-nodes. *Lancet* 1997;**349**:1864–7.

26. Turner RR, Ollila DW, Krasne DL, et al. Histopathologic validation of the sentinel lymph node hypothesis for breast carcinoma. *Ann Surg* 1997;**226**:271–8.

27. Gentry JF. Pelvic lymph node metastases in prostatic carcinoma. The value of touch imprint cytology. *Am J Surg Pathol* 1986;**10**:718–27.

28. Hadjiminas DJ, Burke M. Intraoperative assessment of nodal status in the selection of patients with breast cancer for axillary clearance. *Br J Surg* 1994;**81**:1615–16.

29. Fisher CJ, Boyle S, Burke M, et al. Intraoperative assessment of nodal status in the selection of patients with breast cancer for axillary clearance. *Br J Surg* 1993;**80**:457–8.

30. Motomura K, Inaji H, Komoike Y, et al. Intraoperative sentinel lymph node examination by imprint cytology and frozen sectioning during breast surgery. *Br J Surg* 2000;**87**:597–601.

31. Ratanawichitrasin A, Biscotti CV, Levy L, et al. Touch imprint cytological analysis of sentinel lymph nodes for detecting axillary metastases in patients with breast cancer. *Br J Surg* 1999;**86**:1346–8.

32. Cserni G. The potential value of intraoperative imprint cytology of axillary sentinel lymph nodes in breast cancer patients. *Am Surg* 2001;**67**:86–91.

33. Turner RR, Ollila DW, Stern S, et al. Optimal histopathologic examination of the sentinel lymph node for breast carcinoma staging. *Am J Surg Pathol* 1999;**23**:263– 7.

34. Torrenga H, Rahusen FD, Meijer S, et al. Sentinel node in breast cancer: detailed analysis of the yield from step sectioning and immunohistochemistry. *J Clin Pathol* 2001;**54**:553–5.

35. Torrenga H, Diest PJ van, Meijer S. Sentinel-node biopsy in breast cancer. *Lancet* 2001;**358**:1814.

36. de Hullu JA, Hollema H, Piers DA, et al. Sentinel lymph node procedure is highly accurate in squamous cell carcinoma of the vulva. *J Clin Oncol* 2000;**18**:2811–16.

37. de Hullu JA, Doting E, Piers DA, et al. Sentinel lymph node identification with technetium-99m-labeled nanocolloid in squamous cell cancer of the vulva. *J Nucl Med* 1998;**39**:1381–5.

38. de Hullu JA, Piers DA, Hollema H, et al. Sentinel lymph node detection in locally recurrent carcinoma of the vulva. *Br J Obstet Gynaecol* 2001;**108**:766–8.

39. Levenback C. Intraoperative lymphatic mapping and sentinel node identification: gynecologic applications. *Recent Results Cancer Res* 2000;**157**:150–8.

40. Van den Brekel MWM, Stel HV, van der Valk P, et al. Micrometastases from squamous cell carcinoma in neck dissection specimens. *Eur Arch Otorhinolaryngol* 1992;**249**:349–53.

41. Motomura K, Inaji H, Komoike Y, et al. Gamma probe and ultrasonographically-guided fine-needle aspiration biopsy of sentinel lymph nodes in breast cancer patients. *Eur J Surg Oncol* 2001;**27**:141–5.

42. Joensuu H, Klemi PJ, Eerola E. Flow cytometric DNA analysis combined with fine needle aspiration biopsy in the diagnosis of palpable metastases. *Analy Quant Cytol Histol* 1988;**10**:256–60.

43. Leers M, Schoffelen R, Theunissen P, et al. Multiparameter flow cytometry (MP-FCM) as a tool for the detection of micrometastatic tumour cells in the sentinel lymph node procedure. *J Clin Pathol* 2002;**55**:359–66.

44. Noguchi S, Aihara T, Motomura K, et al. Detection of breast cancer micrometastases in axillary lymph nodes by means of reverse transcriptase-polymerase chain reaction. Comparison between MUC1 mRNA and keratin 19 mRNA amplification. *Am J Pathol* 1996;**148**:649–56.

45. Hoon DSB, Sarantou T, Doi F, et al. Detection of metastatic breast cancer by β-hcg polymerase chain reaction. *Int J Cancer* 1996;**69**:369–74.

46. Schoenfeld A, Luqmani Y, Smith D, et al. Detection of breast cancer micrometastases in axillary lymph nodes by using polymerase chain reaction. *Cancer Res* 1994;**54**:2986–90.

47. Noguchi S, Tomohiko A, Motomura K, et al. Detection of breast cancer micrometastases in axillary lymph nodes by means of reverse transcriptase-polymerase chain reaction. *Cancer* 1994;**74**:1595–600.

48. Kataoka A, Mori M, Sadanaga N, et al. RT-PCR detection of breast cancer cells in sentinel lymph nodes. *Int J Oncol* 2000;**16**:1147–52.

49. Mori M, Mimori K, Inoue H, et al. Detection of cancer micrometastases in lymph nodes by reverse transcriptase-polymerase chain reaction. *Cancer Res* 1995;**55**:3417–20.

50. Wascher RA, Bostick PJ, Huynh KT, et al. Detection of MAGE-A3 in breast cancer patients' sentinel lymph nodes. *Br J Cancer* 2001;**85**:1340–6.

51. Manzotti M, Dell'Orto P, Maisonneuve P, et al. Reverse transcription-polymerase chain reaction assay for multiple mRNA markers in the detection of breast cancer metastases in sentinel lymph nodes. *Int J Cancer* 2001;**95**:307–12.

52. Ishida M, Kitamura K, Kinoshita J, et al. Detection of micrometastasis in the sentinel lymph nodes in breast cancer. *Surgery* 2002;**131**(1 Pt 2):S211–16.

53. Van Trappen PO, Gyselman VG, Lowe DG, et al. Molecular quantification and mapping of lymph-node micrometastases in cervical cancer. *Lancet* 2001;**357**:15–20.

54. Palmieri G, Ascierto PA, Cossu A, et al. Detection of occult melanoma cells in paraffin-embedded histologically negative sentinel lymph nodes using a reverse transcriptase polymerase chain reaction assay. *J Clin Oncol* 2001;**19**:1437–43.

55. Bostick PJ, Chatterjee S, Chi DD, et al. Limitations of specific reverse-transcriptase polymerase chain reaction markers in the detection of metastases in the lymph nodes and blood of breast cancer patients. *J Clin Oncol* 1998;**16**:2632–40.

56. van der Velde-Zimmermann D, Schipper ME, de Weger RA, et al. Sentinel node biopsies in melanoma patients: a protocol for accurate, efficient, and cost-effective analysis by preselection for immunohistochemistry on the basis of Tyr-PCR. *Ann Surg Oncol* 2000;**7**:51–4.

57. Bostick PJ, Huynh KT, Sarantou T, et al. Detection of metastases in sentinel lymph nodes of breast cancer patients by multiple-marker RT-PCR. *Int J Cancer* 1998;**79**:645–51.

58. Cserni G. Metastases in axillary sentinel lymph nodes in breast cancer as detected by intensive histopathological workup. *J Clin Pathol* 1999;**52**:922–4.

59. Zhang PJ, Reisner RM, Nangia R, et al. Effectiveness of multiple level sectioning in detecting axillary nodal micrometastasis in breast cancer. A retrospective study with immunohistochemical analysis. *Arch Pathol Lab Med* 1998;**122**:687–90.

60. Borgstein PJ, Pijpers R, Comans EF, et al. Sentinel lymph node biopsy in breast cancer: guidelines and pitfalls of lymphoscintigraphy and gamma probe detection. *J Am Coll Surg* 1998;**186**:275–83.

61. Borgstein PJ, Meijer S, Pijpers R, et al. Functional lymphatic anatomy for sentinel node biopsy in breast cancer: echoes from the past and the periareolar blue method. *Ann Surg* 2000;**232**:81–9.

62. Pijpers R, Meyer S, Hoekstra OS, et al. Impact of lymphoscintigraphy on sentinel node identification with technetium-99m-colloidal albumin in breast cancer. *J Nucl Med* 1997;**38**:366–8.

63. Pijpers R, Borgstein PJ, Meijer S, et al. Sentinel node biopsy in melanoma patients: dynamic lymphoscintigraphy followed by intraoperative gamma probe and vital blue guidance. *World J Surg* 1997;**21**:788–92.

64. Verheijen RH, Pijpers R, van Diest PJ, et al. Sentinel node detection in cervical cancer. *Obstet Gynecol* 2000;**96**:135–13

65. Dowlatshahi K, Fan M, Bloom KJ, et al. Occult metastases in the sentinel lymph nodes of patients with early stage breast carcinoma: a preliminary study. *Cancer* 1999;**86**:990–6.

66. Rahusen FD, Torrenga H, van Diest PJ, et al. Predictive factors for metastatic involvement of nonsentinel nodes in patients with breast cancer. *Arch Surg* 2001;**136**:1059–63.

67. Turner RR, Chu KU, Qi K, et al. Pathologic features associated with nonsentinel lymph node metastases in patients with metastatic breast carcinoma in a sentinel lymph node. *Cancer* 2000;**89**:574–81.

68. Jannink I, Fan M, Nagy S, et al. Serial sectioning of sentinel nodes in patients with breast cancer: a pilot study. *Ann Surg Oncol* 1998;**5**:310–14.

69. Pendas S, Dauway E, Cox CE, et al. Sentinel node biopsy and cytokeratin staining for the accurate staging of 478 breast cancer patients. *Am Surg* 1999;**65**:500–5.

70. Schreiber RH, Pendas S, Ku NN, et al. Microstaging of breast cancer patients using cytokeratin staining of the sentinel lymph node. *Ann Surg Oncol* 1999;**6**:95–101.

71. Kowolik JH, Kuhn W, Nahrig J, et al. Detection of micrometastases in sentinel lymph nodes of the breast applying monoclonal antibodies AE1/AE3 to pancytokeratins. *Oncol Rep* 2000;**7**:745–9.

72. Hsieh PP, Ho WL, Yeh DC, et al. Histopathologic analysis of sentinel lymph nodes in breast carcinoma. *Zhonghua Yi Xue Za Zhi (Taipei)* 2000;**63**:744–50.

73. Terada KY, Shimizu DM, Wong JH. Sentinel node dissection and ultrastaging in squamous cell cancer of the vulva. *Gynecol Oncol* 2000;**76**:40–4.

74. Mann BG, Buchanan M, Collins PJ, et al. High incidence of micrometastases in breast cancer sentinel nodes. *Aust N Z J Surg* 2000;**70**:786–90.

75. Molpus KL, Kelley MC, Johnson JE, et al. Sentinel lymph node detection and micro-staging in vulvar carcinoma. *J Reprod Med* 2001;**46**:863–9.

5 SENTINEL LYMPH NODE PROCEDURE IN VULVAR CANCER

JA DE HULLU, AND ATE G.J. VAN DER ZEE

INTRODUCTION

Vulvar cancer represents approximately 4% of all gynecologic malignancies. The mean age at presentation of patients with vulvar cancer is about 70 years. Squamous cell carcinomas account for 90% of vulvar cancer cases; melanomas, adenocarcinomas, basal cell carcinomas, and sarcomas account for the rest.[1] This chapter discusses the rationale for the sentinel lymph node procedure in vulvar cancer and provides a step-by-step description of the sentinel lymph node procedure performed with the combination of ^{99m}Tc-labeled nanocolloid and patent blue dye) in patients with squamous cell carcinoma of the vulva. Selection of patients, preoperative care, how and where to inject nanocolloid and dye around the tumor, equipment necessary for the procedure, and details of histopathologic examination are discussed. The literature on sentinel lymph node biopsy in patients with vulvar cancer is reviewed. Finally, a preliminary experience with the sentinel lymph node procedure in patients with melanoma of the vulva is reviewed.

RATIONALE FOR THE SENTINEL LYMPH NODE PROCEDURE IN VULVAR CANCER

Squamous cell carcinoma of the vulva may spread by three routes: direct extension and spread through the lymph channels or blood vessels. Direct extension is infrequent. Initial spread usually occurs through lymph channels to the inguinofemoral lymph nodes. Hematogenous spread is rare in early-stage disease. Since 1988, the staging system for vulvar cancer (Table 5.1) has been based on findings at surgery and on histopathologic review.[2] Stage IA vulvar cancer with a depth of invasion less than 1 mm was added because of the negligible risk of lymph node metastasis.[3,4]

The overall prognosis for patients with vulvar cancer with a depth of invasion greater than 1 mm is good, with 5-year survival rates around 70% since the introduction of radical vulvectomy with en bloc inguinofemoral lymphadenectomy in the early part of the twentieth century.[1] The number of inguinofemoral lymph node metastases is the most important prognostic factor.[1] However, although survival figures are good, the short- and long-term morbidity associated with radical vulvectomy with en bloc inguinofemoral lymphadenectomy is substantial. Eighty-five percent of patients experience a complication

Table 5.1 Staging system for vulvar cancer of the International Federation of Gynecology and Obstetrics (FIGO).

Stage I	Lesions 2 cm or less in size confined to the vulva or perineum. No nodal metastasis.
Stage IA	Lesions 2 cm or less in size confined to the vulva or perineum and with stromal invasion no greater than 1.0 mm.* No nodal metastasis.
Stage II	Tumor confined to the vulva and/or perineum or more than 2 cm in the greatest dimension. No nodal metastasis.
Stage III	Tumor of any size with: (i) Adjacent spread of the lower urethra and/or the vagina or anus, and/or (ii) unilateral regional lymph node metastasis.
Stage IVA	Tumor invades upper urethra, bladder mucosa, rectal mucosa, pelvic bone, and/or bilateral regional node metastasis. or
Stage IVB	Any distant metastasis, including pelvic lymph nodes.

* The depth of invasion is defined as the measurement of the tumor from the epithelial–stromal junction of the adjacent most superficial dermal papilla to the deepest point of invasion.

(infection, lymphocyst, wound breakdown, or lymphedema), and these complications often result in prolonged hospitalization.[5] Psychosexual consequences include dramatic distortions in body image and diminished sexual activity and function.[6]

Since the end of the twentieth century, the generally accepted standard treatment for early-stage vulvar cancer (T1 tumor [diameter $\leq$ 2 cm] or a T2 tumor [diameter > 2 cm] without suspicious lymph nodes at palpation) has been wide local excision with unilateral or bilateral inguinofemoral lymphadenectomy via separate incisions. Radical vulvectomy is performed only in the case of a multifocal tumor. Unilateral inguinofemoral lymphadenectomy is performed when the medial margins of the tumor are more than 1 cm from the midline.[7] Postoperative radiotherapy is given when more than one lymph node contains metastases or any lymph node metastasis is associated with extranodal extension. Treatment for patients with advanced disease—as with bulky lymph nodes or with involvement of the anus, rectum, or urethra—is individualized and usually consists of multimodality treatment (radiotherapy with or without concurrent chemotherapy or surgery).

The practice of performing complete inguinofemoral lymphadenectomy in patients with early-stage disease is based on the assumption that the prognosis is better after elective inguinofemoral lymphadenectomy than it is with surveillance of the groin. However, no randomized trial has addressed the issue of elective versus delayed inguinofemoral lymphadenectomy in patients with vulvar cancer and clinically normal nodes. It is unlikely that such a trial will be performed in the future, as prospects are very poor for patients with vulvar cancer that recurs in an initially untreated groin.[8] A trial by the Gynecologic Oncology Group comparing elective inguinofemoral lymphadenectomy versus elective irradiation of the groin was stopped prematurely because of an increased recurrence rate and a worse outcome for patients in the radiotherapy arm of the trial.[9]

Only 20–30% of patients with early-stage disease have inguinofemoral lymph node metastases. The other 70–80% of patients will probably not benefit from inguinofemoral lymphadenectomy but are at risk from the morbidity of this procedure. Although the introduction of separate incisions has lowered the complication rate compared to the rate seen with the en bloc approach, seroma and lymphedema of the legs are still frequently observed,[10] and tumor recurrences in the skin bridge have occasionally been reported.[10–15]

Unfortunately, at present, no accurate noninvasive techniques are available for the detection of inguinofemoral lymph node metastases. Physical examination (palpation of the groin) is accurate in only 25% of cases.[5] The results of sonography[16] and positron emission tomography[17] in predicting the lymph node status in patients with vulvar cancer are disappointing. No published studies are available about the diagnostic value of computed tomography and magnetic resonance imaging. A promising technique is ultrasound-guided fine-needle biopsy at outpatient visits to detect lymph node metastase.[18] An important issue concerning this technique, however, is that its success rate depends mainly on the experience of the investigator.

The lack of accurate noninvasive techniques for detecting inguinofemoral lymph node metastases in combination with the absence of lymph node metastases in the majority of patients with early-stage disease has led to the development of the minimally invasive sentinel lymph node procedure in vulvar cancer.

SENTINEL LYMPH NODE PROCEDURES IN PATIENTS WITH SQUAMOUS CELL CARCINOMA OF THE VULVA

In this section we describe the sentinel node procedure as performed at the University Hospital Groningen. Each practice setting will have slightly different resources available.

Selection of patients and care until hospital admission

Patients are selected for the sentinel lymph node procedure at their first visit at the outpatient clinic. To be eligible for the sentinel lymph node procedure, patients need to fulfill the following criteria:

1) Histologically proven squamous cell carcinoma of the vulva with depth of invasion greater than 1 mm. When the patient is referred from another hospital, the tissue slides are subjected to histopathologic review. If necessary, punch biopsy is repeated. In general, punch biopsy is preferred to excisional biopsy for diagnosis, because the sentinel lymph node procedure is more accurate with injections around a tumor after a punch biopsy than with injections around a scar after excision.

2) A tumor small enough that injection around the tumor is technically possible. For that reason, patients with tumors larger than 4 cm are excluded from the sentinel lymph node procedure.
3) No fixed lymph nodes in the groins.

At the first outpatient visit, the patient is informed about the different aspects of the sentinel lymph node procedure. It is particularly important to inform the patient that the appearance of sentinel lymph nodes on the lymphoscintigram after injection of [99mTc]-labeled nanocolloid means not that there are metastases but rather that the first part of the sentinel lymph node procedure has been successful. At the end of the first visit, the patient is given a prescription for lidocaine-prilocaine 5% cream (EMLA, Astra Pharmaceuticals, L.P., Westborough, MA, USA) and advised to apply the cream on the vulva at least half an hour before her appointment at the Department of Nuclear Medicine (see the next section).

Lymphoscintigraphy

Two days before operation, in the Department of Nuclear Medicine, 0.5 ml (100 MBq) of [99mTc]-labeled nanocolloid (Solco Nuclear, Birfelden, Switzerland) is prepared for the sentinel lymph node procedure. The gynecologist injects the nanocolloid intradermally at four locations around the tumor using a short needle (25 gauge) (Figures 5.1–5.6). It is important not to spill any nanocolloid on the vulva or the groin, as these tiny droplets will clearly show up on the lymphoscintigram and might make its accurate interpretation difficult. Anterior images are obtained with a single-headed gamma camera with a low-energy, high-resolution collimator. Immediately after injection, dynamic imaging is started.

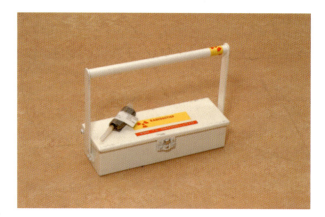

Figure 5.1 Syringe with [99mTc]-labeled radiocolloid.

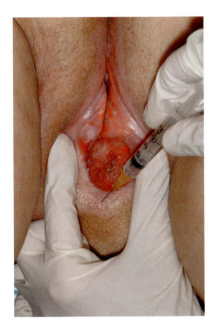

Figure 5.2 Site of injection.

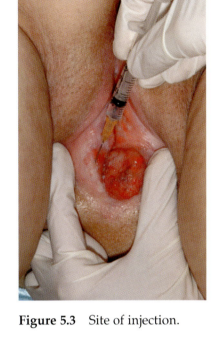

Figure 5.3 Site of injection.

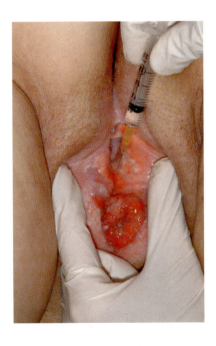

Figure 5.4 Site of injection.

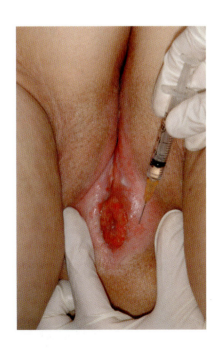

Figure 5.5 Site of injection.

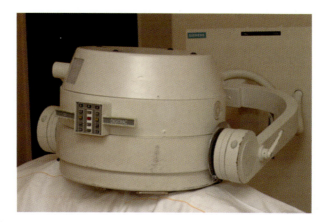

Figure 5.6   Gamma camera.

Thirty-second frames are obtained over the course of 30 min (Figures 5.7 and 5.8). Anterior and lateral static images are obtained 2.5 h after nanocolloid injection. To facilitate interpretation of transmission, scanning is performed simultaneously, using the 120-keV gamma rays of a cobalt-57 flood source. The first-appearing persistent focal accumulation along each lymphatic channel is considered to be a sentinel lymph node. The sites of the sentinel lymph nodes are marked on the skin with a pencil by the nuclear medicine physician. Marks showing the locations of sentinel lymph nodes are shown in Figure 5.9. The lymphoscintigram should be available during the operation the next day.

Notification of pathologist before surgery

The day before operation, the pathologist should be informed about the planned operation in order to prepare for frozen-section analysis of the sentinel lymph nodes.

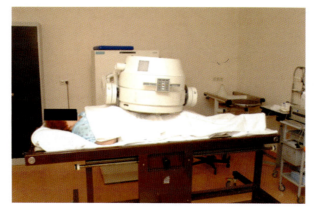

Figure 5.7   Position of the patient during dynamic scanning.

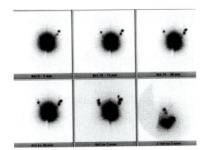

Figure 5.8 Uptake of radionuclide in patient with a midline lesion and multiple bilateral sentinel nodes. These scans do not conclusively show which of these nodes are sentinel and which are second-echelon. Extensive uptake of radionuclide to second-echelon nodes in the pelvic, common iliac, and low para-aortic lymph nodes in a patient with a vulvar cancer on the left close to the midline.

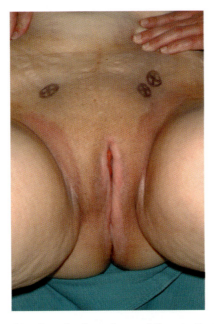

Figure 5.9 Marks on the skin indicating the locations of the sentinel lymph nodes.

Operation

On the day of surgery, after induction of anesthesia, stirrups are used to secure the lower extremities with the knees bent at right angles and the legs separated (Figure 5.10). The hips are not flexed during the sentinel lymph node procedure. The bladder is catheterized. A digital photograph is made of the tumor. Two milliliters of patent blue-V (2.5% in aqueous solution containing 0.6% sodium chloride and 0.05% disodium hydrogen phosphate; Laboratoire Guerbet, Aulney-Sous-Bois, France) is injected at four locations around the tumor (Figure 5.11). A hand-held gamma-ray detection probe (Neoprobe, Neoprobe Corp., Dublin, OH, USA) is used to confirm that the marks drawn on the skin after lymphoscintigraphy correspond to the areas of greatest activity in the groin (Figures 5.12–5.15). It is our experience that the 'hot spots' as found with the hand-held probe are often about 1 cm distal from where the nuclear medicine physician has marked the skin, probably because of different positioning of the patient during lymphoscintigraphy and during surgery. During the learning curve of the sentinel lymph node procedure (at least 10 cases), it may be helpful to invite the nuclear medicine physician to be in the operating theater to assist in identifying the sentinel lymph nodes. A small skin incision (3–4 cm) is

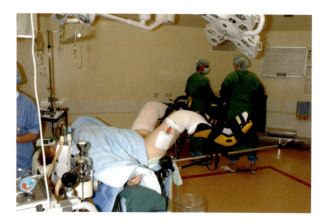

Figure 5.10   Position of the patient during the sentinel lymph node procedure.

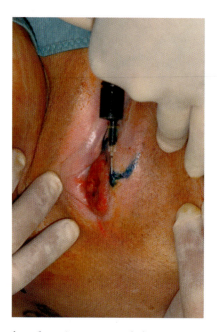

Figure 5.11   Injection of blue dye at four locations around the tumor.

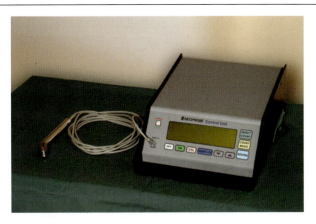

Figure 5.12   Hand-held gamma probe.

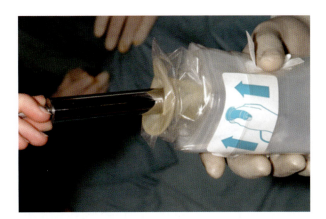

Figure 5.13   Plastic bag for sterile use of the probe.

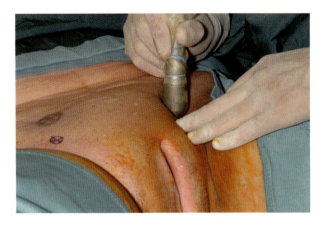

Figure 5.14   Confirmation of the site with the highest radioactivity.

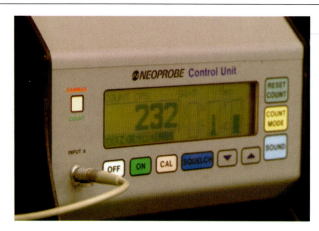

Figure 5.15   Counts of radioactivity.

made below each marked spot, and the sentinel lymph nodes are identified with use of the hand-held probe and careful dissection of blue-stained vessels (Figures 5.16–5.19).

Immediately after removal, sentinel lymph nodes are sent for frozen-section examination (Figure 5.20). In general, the sensitivity of frozen-section examination in the detection of metastases is about 80%. The advantage of frozen-section examination is that patients with a positive sentinel lymph node at frozen section can undergo an immediate lymphadenectomy instead of a second procedure. After removal of sentinel lymph nodes, the wound bed is re-examined for residual radioactivity, and if the level of residual radioactivity is more than 10% of the radioactivity level of the first sentinel lymph node, the search for sentinel lymph nodes is continued (Figure 5.21). When the search for sentinel lymph nodes in the first groin takes more than about 20 min, the patent blue can disappear from sentinel nodes and spread to other, second-echelon and even higher-up lymph nodes. In this situation, patent blue is reinjected before exploration of the other groin to maximize the opportunity for finding blue lymph nodes in the second groin.

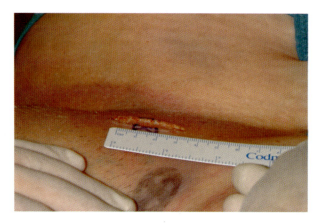

Figure 5.16   Small incision in the skin over site with high radioactivity.

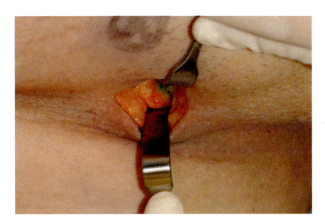

Figure 5.17   Blue lymph vessel.

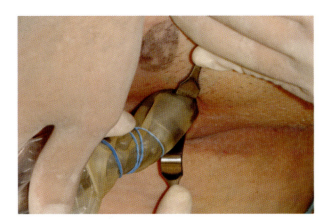

Figure 5.18   Checking the point of highest radioactivity.

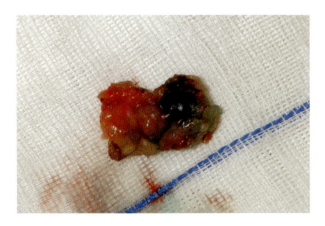

Figure 5.19   Removed blue lymph node.

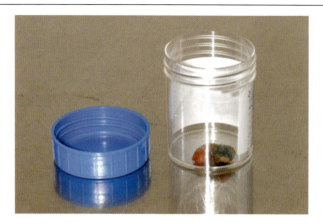

Figure 5.20   Blue lymph node is sent for frozen-section examination.

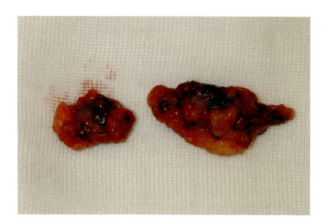

Figure 5.21   Additional sentinel lymph node identified because of residual radioactivity.

After completion of the sentinel lymph node procedure, the primary tumor is removed by wide local excision (Figure 5.22). (As mentioned earlier, modified radical vulvectomy is performed in the case of a multifocal tumor or an abnormal aspect of the vulva.) Removal of the primary tumor together with the sites where nanocolloid was injected decreases background radiation levels in the groins. For that reason, the groins are checked for additional sentinel lymph nodes after excision of the primary tumor. Moreover, when at the start of the operation it appears impossible to identify 'hot spots' in the groin with the hand-held probe, it is often helpful to remove the primary tumor first.

When metastatic disease is detected in frozen sections of the sentinel lymph nodes, complete inguinofemoral lymphadenectomy is performed in the groin(s) with metastastic disease.

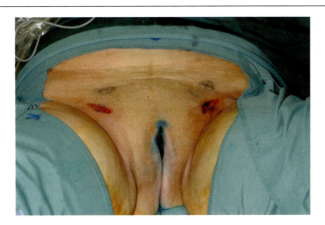

Figure 5.22   Overview of the incisions after sentinel lymph node procedure.

Pathologic examination of lymph nodes

As mentioned earlier, before the sentinel lymph node procedure is started, the pathologist is informed about the planned procedure. For sentinel nodes in which metastases are found on frozen-section examination and for routine histopathologic examination of all other lymph nodes, one section per 0.5 cm of the node is cut and stained with hematoxylin-eosin (HE). For sentinel lymph nodes in which no metastases are found on frozen-section examination, additional pairs of sections are subsequently cut with three sections/mm. One section of each pair is stained with HE, and the other section is immunostained with cytokeratin 1% AE1:AE3 antikeratin solution (Boehringer Mannheim, Mannheim, Germany). Van Diest et al[19] advise cutting additional pairs of sections of sentinel lymph nodes after lamellating the nodes into pieces of 0.5 cm; five steps with 250 μm: interval, one section stained with HE, and the other immunostained. The optimal policy for ultrastaging is not known at present (see also Chapter 4, 'Ultrastaging of the sentinel node'). A compromise should be found between sensitivity and workload. When micrometastases are detected on immunohistochemical analysis, unilateral or bilateral inguinofemoral lymphadenectomy has to be performed in a second operation.

LITERATURE ON SENTINEL LYMPH NODE PROCEDURE IN VULVAR CANCER

In vulvar cancer, DiSaia et al were the first to postulate that the superficial groin nodes might serve as sentinel lymph nodes.[20] These authors performed frozen-section examination of the superficial groin nodes and carried out complete inguinofemoral lymphadenectomy only when metastastic disease was found at frozen section. However, in later studies, femoral lymph node metastases were reported after biopsy of tumor-free superficial inguinal lymph nodes.[21]

In 1994, Levenback et al published the first feasibility study of the sentinel lymph node procedure with isosulfan blue in nine patients with vulvar cancer (two melanomas and seven squamous cell carcinomas).[22] After the sentinel lymph node procedure, complete inguinofemoral lymphadenectomy via separate incisions was performed. Sentinel lymph nodes were identified in seven of 12 groins. No complications were observed, and the disease status of the sentinel lymph nodes appeared to be representative of the disease status of the nonsentinel lymph nodes. This experience was extended to 21 patients in 1995 and 52 patients in 2001.[23,24]

In 1997, DeCesare et al[25] published results of a feasibility study on the sentinel lymph node procedure with intraoperative gamma ray detection, and de Hullu et al[26] published results achieved using the combined technique (preoperative lymphoscintigraphy and intraoperative patent blue). Both techniques were feasible.

Once it had been shown that the sentinel lymph node procedure was feasible, further investigations were necessary to analyze whether the accuracy of the procedure was high enough to justify incorporation of the technique into routine clinical practice. Patients with groin recurrence can rarely be treated successfully with salvage therapy; therefore, the false-negative sentinel node rate must be very low to be acceptable to patients and clinicians. In most of these studies, sentinel lymph node identification was followed by a full confirmative inguinofemoral lymphadenectomy.

In 1999, Ansink et al[27] published the first large series of patients with vulvar cancer in whom the negative predictive value of the sentinel lymph node procedure was investigated. In this multicenter study, only blue dye was used. Sentinel lymph nodes were identified in 56% of the patients, and a false-negative sentinel lymph node was found in two of 51 patients. In interpreting the sentinel lymph node identification rate of only 56%, one has to keep in mind that this was a multicenter study that included surgeons at the beginning of the learning curve. Moreover, of the six centers that participated in the study, three contributed six or fewer patients; 80% of the patients came from two centers. Levenback et al[24] reported an identification rate of 88% in a group of 52 patients who underwent lymphatic mapping with blue dye alone. Early in the study, there were two patients with positive nodes in whom a sentinel node was not identified. The learning curve may have played an important role in the technical success rate in both the Ansink and Levenback studies. Shortly after this publication, De Cicco et al[28] reported no false-negative sentinel lymph nodes in 37 patients who underwent preoperative lymphoscintigraphy and gamma-probe-guided surgery. De Hullu et al[26] used the combined technique and reported no false-negative sentinel lymph nodes in 59 patients. In the de Hullu et al study, no false-negative sentinel lymph nodes were found with either preoperative or intraoperative use of a radioactive tracer.

It is remarkable that two centers have published about the sentinel lymph node procedure as part of the standard treatment for vulvar cancer.[29,30] In 1999, Rodier et al reported the results of the sentinel lymph node procedure with the combined technique in eight patients.[29] Complete inguinofemoral lymphadenectomy was performed only in the case of a positive sentinel lymph node (one patient) or an unsuccessful procedure (failure to detect a sentinel lymph node; one patient). The follow-up time for the six patients with negative sentinel nodes ranged from only 1 month to 7 months, too short to permit conclusion regarding whether this option is safe. In 2000, Terada et al summarized their experience with nine patients who underwent the sentinel lymph node procedure as standard nodal staging.[30] Initially, the sentinel lymph nodes were bivalved and examined after routine HE staining. Only one patient had nodal metastases, and in this patient a complete inguinofemoral lymphadenectomy was subsequently performed. No further metastases were found at complete lymphadenectomy. Later, this patient developed a recurrence in the opposite groin. As a result of this recurrence, the protocol for pathologic examination of sentinel lymph nodes was changed to ultrastaging (lateral sectioning of the sentinel lymph nodes at 3-mm intervals and then cutting of each block at 40-μm intervals). On ultrastaging performed after recurrence in the one patient who experienced a groin recurrence, the sentinel lymph node in the groin with the lymph node recurrence was found to contain a micrometastasis. Finally, two (14%) of 14 sentinel lymph nodes negative by conventional staining were positive on ultrastaging. Although the Rodier et al and Terada et al studies are interesting pilot studies, it is our opinion that at the time these studies were performed, experience with the sentinel lymph node procedure was not mature enough to justify its use as the standard procedure for nodal staging. These centers did not report their learning curves and did not participate in clinical trials sufficiently powered to permit evaluation of the safety of the sentinel lymph node procedure in vulvar cancer.

An extensive study has been started in the USA (Gynecologic Oncology Group trial 173) to determine the validity of the sentinel lymph node procedure in vulvar cancer. The ideal population in which to investigate the accuracy of the sentinel lymph node procedure is patients with at least a moderate likelihood of clinically occult nodal metastases. To increase the proportion of patients with lymph node metastases, only patients with tumors of at least 2 cm are eligible for inclusion in the study.

Table 5.2 summarizes all of the series published to date regarding lymphatic mapping in patients with vulvar cancer. In the majority of patients, the sentinel lymph node procedure was followed by standard unilateral or bilateral inguinofemoral lymphadenectomy via separate incisions. The technical success rate of 95.8% by patient is excellent. The success rate by groin is much lower; however, we must recall that in most patients bilateral groin dissections were performed if the lesion was close to the midline. Some of these patients probably had only unilateral lymphatic drainage. For these combined series, the sensitivity is 96.5% and the negative predictive value is 98.7%. Interestingly, extended histologic evaluation of sentinel lymph nodes revealed micrometastases missed by conventional HE staining in only 6.4% of cases, much lower than the proportion in breast cancer and melanoma patients.

Table 5.2 Published studies of lymphatic mapping and sentinel node identification in patients with vulvar cancer.

Investigator, Year, Reference	Technique	Technical Success, Patients	Technical Success, Groins	Specificity	Sensitivity	NPV	Accuracy	SN Only + LN/groin	Node + technical failures (groin)	Micro mets on serial sections
Barton, 1992[47]	Preop LS	9/10	13/16	6/6	3/3	6/6	9/9	1/3	1	–
DeCesar, 1997[25]	Intraop LS	11/11	17/17	8/8	3/3	8/8	11/11	1/4	0	–
Rodier, 1999[29]	Multiple techniques	7/8	8/10	7/7	1/1	7/7	7/7	1/1	0	–
Echt, 1999[42]	Blue dye	9/12	13/23	6/6	2/2	6/6	8/8	2/3	1	–
Ansink, 1999[27]	Blue dye	n/a	52/93	41/41	9/11	41/43	50/52	6/14	1	–
Sideri, 2000[28]	Preop LS Intraop LS	44/44	77/77	31/31	13/13	31/31	44/44	10/13	1	–
Terada, 2000*[30]	PreopLS Intraop LS Blue dye	10/10	12/12	8/8	1/2	8/9	9/10	2/2	0	1/15
de Hullu, 2000[26]	Preop LS Intraop LS Blue dye	59/59	95/107	39/39	20/20	39/39	59/59	15/27	0	4/102
Molpus, 2001[43]	Preop LS Intraop LS Blue dye	11/11	13/16	9/9	2/2	9/9	11/11	1/3	1	–
Tavares, 2001[44]	Preop LS Intraop LS Blue dye	15/15	n/a	12/12	3/3	12/12	15/15	2/3	0	
Levenback, 2001[24]	Blue dye	– 46/52	57/76	37/37	9/9	37/37	46/46	6/11	2	–
Sliutz, 2002[46]	Preop LS Intraop LS	26/26	46/46	17/17	9/9	17/17	26/26	n/a	0	–

Table 5.2 cont.

Investigator, Year, Reference	Technique	Technical Success, Patients	Technical Success, Groins	Specificity	Sensitivity	NPV	Accuracy	SN Only + LN/groin	Node + technical failures (groin)	Micro mets on serial sections
Puig-Tintore, 2003[45]	Preop LS Intraop LS Blue dye	25/26	31/39	17/17	8/8	17/17	25/25	6/9	1	3/8
Total		272/284 (95.8)	434/532 (81.6)	238/238 (100)	83/86 (96.5)	238/241 (98.7)	320/323 (99)	53/93 (57)	8	8/125 (6.4)

✓Technical success: number of patients or groins in which SLNs were found at surgery/total number of patients or groins.

✓ Sensitivity: proportion of patients with groin metastases in whom the SLNs contained tumor (true positive/[true positive + false negative]).

Negative predictive value (NPV): proportion of patients without tumor in SLNs in whom the groin was free of tumor (true negative/[true negative + false negative]).

✓ Accuracy: proportion of patients with successful SLN biopsy in whom the status of the SLN correlated with the status of the groin ([true positive + true negative]/[true positive + true negative + false positive + false negative]).

Preop: preoperative; LS: lymphoscintigraphy; intraop: intraoperative; micro mets: micrometastases; SLN: sentinel node.

*Full lymphadenectomy was only performed in case of positive sentinel node.

SENTINEL LYMPH NODE PROCEDURE IN VULVAR MELANOMA

Vulvar melanoma is the second most common vulvar malignancy.[1,31] In contrast with women with cutaneous melanomas, who tend to present at a young age (mean age 35 years) and have 5-year survival rates up to 80%,[32–34] women with vulvar melanomas tend to present at an advanced age (mean age 65 years) and have a 5-year survival rate of only 47% in the largest reported series. Surgery is the only effective therapy for local control of vulvar melanoma. The role of elective lymphadenectomy in vulvar melanoma is controversial. We recently published an overview of our experience with nine patients with vulvar melanoma who underwent the sentinel lymph node procedure according to the protocol described earlier in this chapter.[35] Complete inguinofemoral lymphadenectomy was performed only in the case of a positive sentinel lymph node. Table 5.3 shows the identification rates and results of pathologic examination of sentinel lymph nodes. All sentinel lymph nodes negative at routine histopathologic examination were also negative at step-sectioning and immunohistochemical examination with S-100 and HMB-45. Figures 5.23 and 5.24 show the tumor and the lymphoscintigram, respectively, of patient 3, who had a vulvar melanoma on the clitoris. The sentinel lymph nodes in both groins were negative.

In three patients, the sentinel lymph node was positive.[26] In these groins, subsequent complete inguinofemoral lymphadenectomy was performed. In one of the three patients with positive sentinel lymph nodes, histopathologic examination showed one additional intranodal metastasis. During follow-up, two of nine patients developed groin recurrences. Review of histopathologic examination confirmed absence of pre-existing lymph node tissue in the groin, indicating in-transit metastases. Both patients underwent salvage inguinofemoral lymphadenectomy for locoregional control. At this writing, one patient is without evidence of disease 29 months after groin recurrence. The other patient died of distant metastases. The results for these nine patients were compared with the results for

Table 5.3 Localization of the tumors, identification of the SLNs, and the results of histopathologic examination in nine patients.

Localization of the tumor	Sentinel lymph nodes		Number of metastases
	Left side	Right side	
Clitoris	1	1	0
Clitoris	2	1	0
Clitoris	2	1	0
Right labium	0	2	1
Left labium	1	2	0
Clitoris	1	0	0
Left labium	1	0	0
Urethra	1	1	1
Clitoris	1	1	1

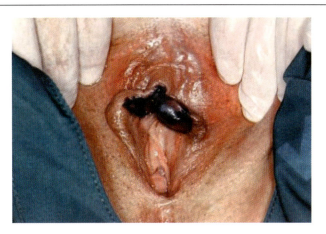

Figure 5.23 Vulvar melanoma.

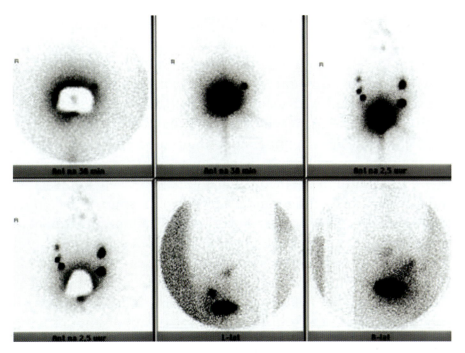

Figure 5.24 Lymphoscintigram of patient with vulvar melanoma. The frames after 30 min show a clear sentinel node on the left side. The frames (with and without central shielding) after 2.5 h show the sentinel node and second echelon nodes on the left side, while on the right side several hot spots are observed. It remains uncertain which hot spot is the sentinel node on the right side. At operation those hot nodes that are also blue will be removed.

24 patients who were treated with radical vulvectomy and complete inguinofemoral lymphadenectomy at our institution. It was concluded that the sentinel lymph node procedure is capable of identifying patients who have clinically occult lymph node metastases and thus may benefit from lymphadenectomy.[26] However, current results also indicate a possible greater risk of in-transit metastases. The sentinel lymph node procedure in patients with vulvar melanoma should be performed only within the context of clinical trials.

GENERAL CONCLUSIONS AND CLINICAL IMPLEMENTATION OF THE SENTINEL LYMPH NODE PROCEDURE IN VULVAR CANCER

The sentinel lymph node procedure appears to be a promising new diagnostic tool for predicting lymph node status in patients with vulvar cancer. The procedure has a very high negative predictive value. Because of the low incidence of squamous cell carcinoma of the vulva, no data are yet available about the safety of omitting inguinofemoral lymphadenectomy in patients with negative sentinel nodes. In speculating about the future role of the sentinel lymph node procedure in vulvar cancer patients, it is useful to consider the present role of this procedure in cutaneous melanoma and breast cancer, two malignancies in which, owing to their relatively high incidences, there is more experience with the sentinel lymph node procedure.

For years, the role of elective lymphadenectomy in patients with cutaneous melanoma with invasion greater then 1 mm has been an issue among surgeons. Four randomized trials failed to demonstrate any survival advantage after elective regional lymphadenectomy.[36] Therefore, the sentinel lymph node procedure was considered an interesting alternative to traditional nodal staging. Essner et al showed no difference in survival between patients treated with elective lymphadenectomy and those treated with the sentinel lymph node procedure,[37] whereas Clary et al found a higher rate of nodal recurrence in patients with a negative sentinel node than in patients without lymph node metastasis at elective inguinofemoral lymphadenectomy.[38] While the diagnostic utility of the sentinel lymph node procedure in cutaneous melanoma has been well established, its therapeutic value and safety in this setting remain unproven. In spite of this, in many centers, the sentinel lymph node procedure is already part of the standard treatment for patients with cutaneous melanoma. To evaluate the possible benefit of the sentinel lymph node procedure, the Multicentre Selective Lymphadenectomy Trial was initiated by Morton.[39] In this phase III study, patients with cutaneous melanoma at least 1 mm thick or with Clark level of at least IV are randomized to wide local excision only or wide local excision with the sentinel lymph node procedure. Only in the case of a positive sentinel lymph node is complete lymphadenectomy performed.[39]

The sentinel lymph node concept has also been developed extensively in breast cancer in the last 10 years. High diagnostic accuracy of the sentinel node procedure in predicting the lymph node status in the axilla has been reported in several studies. Giuliano et al observed 67 patients with a negative sentinel lymph node and found no local or axillary recurrences.[40] In breast cancer patients with a positive sentinel node, it is not clear yet whether further axillary staging gives a survival advantage. There may be a role for postoperative radiotherapy, possibly with chemotherapy, instead of a complete lymphadenectomy. At present, two study groups in the USA are investigating several important issues with respect to the safety, morbidity, and survival outcomes of the sentinel lymph node procedure, complete lymphadenectomy, and radiotherapy in breast cancer patients.[41] In addition, the European Organization for Research and Treatment of Cancer has initiated the

After Mapping of the Axilla Radiotherapy or Surgery protocol, in which patients with a positive sentinel node are randomized to complete axillary dissection or radiotherapy.

To explore further the application of the sentinel lymph node procedure in vulvar cancer, a so-called two-step randomized multicenter study has been designed. In step 1, participating centers will perform sentinel lymph node procedures with subsequent complete inguinofemoral lymphadenectomy in 10 patients as part of the learning curve. When a center has successfully completed step 1, subsequent patients with a negative sentinel lymph node will be randomly assigned to complete inguinofemoral lymphadenectomy or observation in step 2. Primary endpoints in this study will be groin recurrence and quality of life. A major drawback of such a study design is the large number of patients with vulvar cancer needed (approximately 560). Histopathologic techniques such as step-sectioning and immunohistochemistry should be included in the study to find out whether micrometastases have clinical value.

As the start of this randomized trial is awaited, an observational multicenter study with stopping rules has been initiated. Centers are allowed to participate when the learning curve of 10 cases has been finished. Complete inguinofemoral lymphadenectomy is performed only in the case of a positive sentinel lymph node. Patients with negative sentinel lymph node(s) are observed every 2 months. It will be important to take into account the results from this ongoing study in the design of future randomized trials.

In the setting of melanoma of the vulva, the extremely low incidence of this disease means that future study of the lymphatic mapping procedure will be very difficult. In light of the two groin recurrences after findings of negative sentinel lymph nodes and reports in the literature of nodal recurrences after findings of negative sentinel lymph nodes in patients with cutaneous melanoma, a multicenter observational study should be started in patients with vulvar melanoma to determine whether there is any place for the sentinel lymph node procedure in patients with this disease.

SUMMARY

Vulvar cancer is an excellent target for the lymphatic mapping strategy. Multiple single-institution feasibility trials suggest that a high rate of sentinel lymph node identification can be achieved, especially with the combined technique. Progress in this disease site is slowed by the low incidence of cases and by the need for a very low false-negative rate. Gynecologic oncologists are encouraged to perform lymphatic mapping to allow extended pathologic analysis of sentinel lymph nodes and to develop their own technical skills. Some common-sense suggestions for reducing the learning curve for gynecologic oncologists learning the sentinel lymph node procedure are listed in Table 5.4. The sentinel node procedure alone cannot be considered the standard of care for patients with vulvar cancer until further data are collected regarding the safety of this approach.

Table 5.4 Common-sense suggestions for reducing the learning curve for lymphatic mapping for gynecologic oncologists.

- Read descriptions of various procedures
- Perform a lymphatic mapping procedure in an animal laboratory
- Select the technique you will use
- Observe melanoma and breast lymphatic mapping cases
- Invite a surgical oncologist to observe or assist with localization of sentinel nodes
- Select patients carefully
- Perform completion lymphadenectomy to determine your own success rate and false-negative rate

REFERENCES

1. Hacker N, Vulvar cancer. In: Berek J, Hacker N, eds, *Practical Gynecologic Oncology* (Williams & Wilkins: Baltimore, MD, 2000) 553–96.

2. FIGO. Gynecologic staging by the International Federation of Gynecologists and Obstetricians. *Gynecol Oncol* 1989;**35**:125–7.

3. Shepherd J. Staging announcement. FIGO staging of gynecologic cancers, cervical, and vulva. *Int J Gynecol Cancer* 1995;**5**:319.

4. Wilkinson EJ, Rico MJ, Pierson KK. Microinvasive carcinoma of the vulva. *Int J Gynecol Pathol* 1982;**1**:29–39.

5. Podratz KC, Symmonds RE, Taylor WF, et al. Carcinoma of the vulva: analysis of treatment and survival. *Obstet Gynecol* 1983;**61**:63–74.

6. Andersen BL, Hacker NF. Psychosexual adjustment after vulvar surgery. *Obstet Gynecol* 1983;**62**:457–62.

7. Burger M, Hollema H, Bouma J. The side of groin node metastases in unilateral vulvar carcinoma. *Int J Gynecol Cancer* 1996;**6**:318–22.

8. Hacker NF, Nieberg RK, Berek JS, et al. Superficially invasive vulvar cancer with nodal metastases. *Gynecol Oncol* 1983;**15**:65–77.

9. Stehman FB, Bundy BN, Thomas G, et al. Groin dissection versus groin radiation in carcinoma of the vulva: a Gynecologic Oncology Group study. *Int J Radiat Oncol Biol Phys* 1992;**24**:389–96.

10. Hacker NF, Leuchter RS, Berek JS, et al. Radical vulvectomy and bilateral inguinal lymphadenectomy through separate groin incisions. *Obstet Gynecol* 1981;**58**:574–9.

11. Schulz MJ, Penalver M. Recurrent vulvar carcinoma in the intervening tissue bridge in early invasive stage I disease treated by radical vulvectomy and bilateral groin dissection through separate incisions. *Gynecol Oncol* 1989;**35**:383–6.

12. Grimshaw RN, Murdoch JB, Monaghan JM. Radical vulvectomy and bilateral inguinal—femoral lymphadenectomy through separate incisions—experience with 100 cases. *Int J Gynecol Cancer* 1993;**3**:18–23.

13. Christopherson W, Buchsbaum HJ, Voet R, et al. Radical vulvectomy and bilateral groin lymphadenectomy utilizing separate groin incisions: report of a case with recurrence in the intervening skin bridge. *Gynecol Oncol* 1985;**21**:247–51.

14. Rose P. Skin bridge recurrences in vulvar cancer: frequency and management. *Int J Gynecol Cancer* 1999;**9**:508–11.

15. Hopkins M, Reid GC, Morley GW. Radical vulvectomy. The decision for the incision. *Cancer* 1993;**72**:799–803.

16. Makela P, Leminen A, Kaariainen M, et al. Pretreatment sonographic evaluation of inguinal lymph nodes in patients with vulvar malignancy. *J Ultrasound Med* 1993;**5**:255–8.

17. de Hullu J, Pruim J, Que TH, et al. Noninvasive detection of inguinofemoral lymph node metastases in squamous cell cancer (SCC) of the vulva by L-[1-^{11}C]-tyrosine positron emission tomography. *Int J Gynecol Cancer* 1999;**9**:141–6.

18. Abang-Mohammed DK, Uberoi R, de B Lopes A, et al. Inguinal node status by ultrasound in vulva cancer. *Gynecol Oncol* 2000;**77**:93–6.

19. van Diest PJ. Histopathological workup of sentinel lymph nodes: how much is enough? *J Clin Pathol* 1999;**52**:871–3.

20. DiSaia PJ, Creasman WT, Rich WM. An alternate approach to early cancer of the vulva. *Am J Obstet Gynecol* 1979;**133**:825–32.

21. Chu J, Tamimi HK, Figge DC. Femoral node metastases with negative superficial inguinal nodes in early vulvar cancer. *Am J Obstet Gynecol* 1981;**140**:337–9.

22. Levenback C, Burke TW, Gershenson DM, et al. Intraoperative lymphatic mapping for vulvar cancer. *Obstet Gynecol* 1994;**84**:163–7.

23. Levenback C, Burke TW, Morris M, et al. Potential applications of intraoperative lymphatic mapping in vulvar cancer. *Gynecol Oncol* 1995;**59**:216–20.

24. Levenback C, Coleman RL, Burke TW, et al. Intraoperative lymphatic mapping and sentinel node identification with blue dye in patients with vulvar cancer. *Gynecol Oncol* 2001;**83**:276–81.

25. DeCesar SL, Fiorica JV, Roberts WS, et al. A pilot study utilizing intraoperative lymphoscintigraphy for identification of the sentinel lymph nodes in vulvar cancer. *Gynecol Oncol* 1997;**66**:425–8.

26. de Hullu JA, Hollema H, Piers DA, et al. Sentinel lymph node procedure is highly accurate in squamous cell carcinoma of the vulva. *J Clin Oncol* 2000;**18**:2811–16.

27. Ansink AC, Sie-Go DM, van der Velden J, et al. Identification of sentinel lymph nodes in vulvar carcinoma patients with the aid of a patent blue V injection: a multicenter study. *Cancer* 1999;**86**:652–6.

28. Sideri M, De Cicco C, Maggioni A, et al. Detection of sentinel nodes by lymphoscintigraphy and gamma probe guided surgery in vulvar neoplasia. *Tumori* 2000;**86**:359–363.

29. Rodier JF, Janser JC, Routiot T, et al. Sentinel node biopsy in vulvar malignancies: a preliminary feasibility study. *Oncol Rep* 1999;**6**:1249–52.

30. Terada K, Shimizu D, Wong J. Sentinel node dissection and ultrastaging in squamous cell cancer of the vulva. *Gynecol Oncol* 2000;**76**:40–4.

31. Dunton CJ, Kautzky M, Hanau C. Malignant melanoma of the vulva: a review. *Obstet Gynecol Surv* 1995;**50**:739–46.

32. Ragnarsson-Oldin B, Johansson H, Rutqvist LE, et al. Malignant melanoma of the vulva and vagina. Trends in incidence, age distribution, and long-term survival among 245 consecutive cases in Sweden 1960–1984. *Cancer* 1993;**71**:1893–7.

33. Ragnarsson-Olding BK, Nilsson BR, Kanter-Lewensohn LR, et al. Malignant melanoma of the vulva in a nationwide, 25-year study of 219 Swedish females: clinical observations and histopathologic features. *Cancer* 1999;**86**:1273–84.

34. Verones U, Adamus J, Bandiera DC, et al. Delayed regional lymph node dissection in stage I melanoma of the skin of the lower extremities. *Cancer* 1982;**49**:2420–30.

35. de Hullu JA, Hollema H, Hoekstra HJ, et al. Vulvar melanoma: is there a role for sentinel lymph node biopsy? *Cancer* 2002;**94**:486–91.

36. Essner R, Morton DL. Does the tumor status of the regional lymph nodes really matter in melanoma? *Ann Surg Onco* 2001;**8**:749–51.

37. Essner R, Conforti A, Kelley MC, et al. Efficacy of lymphatic mapping, sentinel lymphadenectomy, and selective complete lymph node dissection as a therapeutic procedure for early-stage melanoma. *Ann Surg Oncol* 1999;**6**:442–9.

38. Clary BM, Mann B, Brady MS, et al. Early recurrence after lymphatic mapping and sentinel node biopsy in patients with primary extremity melanoma: a comparison with elective lymph node dissection. *Ann Surg Oncol* 2001;**8**:328–37.

39. Morton DL. Lymphatic mapping and sentinel lymphadenectomy for melanoma: past, present, and future. *Ann Surg Oncol* 2001;**8**:22S–8.

40. Giuliano AE, Haigh PI, Brennan MB, et al. Prospective observational study of sentinel lymphadenectomy without further axillary dissection in patients with sentinel node-negative breast cancer. *J Clin Oncol* 2000;**18**:2553–9.

41. Ross MI. Sentinel node dissection in early-stage breast cancer: ongoing prospective randomized trials in the USA. *Ann Surg Oncol* 2001;**8**:77S–81S.

42. Echt ML, Finan MA, Hoffman MS, et al. Detection of sentinel lymph nodes with lymphazurin in cervical, uterine, and vulvar malignancies. *South Med J* 1999;**92**:204–8.

43. Molpus KL, Kelley MC, Johnson JE, et al. Sentinel lymph node detection and microstaging in vulvar carcinoma. *J Reprod Med* 2001;**46**:863–9.

44. Tavares MG, Sapienza MT, Galeb NA Jr, et al. The use of ^{99m}Tc-phytate for sentinel node mapping in melanoma, breast cancer and vulvar cancer: a study of 100 cases. *Eur J Nucl Med* 2001;**28**:1597–604.

45. Puig-Tintore LM, Ordi J, Vidal-Sicart S, et al. Further data on the usefulness of sentinel lymph node identification and ultrastaging in vulvar squamous cell carcinoma. *Gynecol Oncol* 2003;**88**:29–34.

46. Sliutz G, Reinthaller A, Lantzsch T, et al. Lymphatic mapping of sentinel nodes in early vulvar cancer. *Gynecol Oncol* 2002;**84**:449–52.

47. Barton DPJ, Berman C, Cavanagh D, et al. Lymposcintigraphy in vulvar cancer: a pilot study. *Gynecol Oncol* 1992;**46**:341–344.

6 SENTINEL LYMPH NODE MAPPING IN CERVIX CANCER

ROBERT COLEMAN AND CHARLES LEVENBACK

BACKGROUND

The history of the treatment of cervix cancer is linked to some of the most important advances in oncology in the twentieth century. Cervix cancer was the first solid tumor cured by radiotherapy. In the 1920s, the fundamentals of brachytherapy for cervix cancer were developed. The cervix is a relatively radioresistant organ, and the uterus and vagina can be used to hold instruments loaded with radioactive sources very close to the primary tumor. Because of the inverse square law, which states that dose drops off at a rate of one divided by the square of the distance from a point source, the dose to the bladder and rectum with brachytherapy is tolerable.

Radical surgery for various solid tumors took hold at the start of the twentieth century. Radical hysterectomy was first performed in North America in 1895 and soon became a popular alternative to radiotherapy for patients with early cervix cancer. Surgery avoids all of the late radiation morbidity to the vagina, bladder, and rectum and spares ovarian function in younger patients. Many advances in critical care, blood banking, and antimicrobial therapy have increased the safety of radical hysterectomy over the past century; however, the fundamentals of the operation have not changed much since the most early descriptions.

The incidence and mortality rates for cervix cancer vary widely throughout the world. Incidence and mortality rates for cervix cancer in North America and Europe have dropped by at least 70% since mass screening with the Pap smear was introduced in the 1940s. The incidence of invasive cervix cancer declined from over 32 per 100 000 white women in the 1940s to less than 8 in the 1990s.[1] Incidence and mortality leveled off in the 1990s. The incidence of cervix cancer and mortality rates for this disease continue to be higher among North American blacks, Hispanics, and Native Americans than among whites and Asians. Although the exact cause of this disparity is unknown, the persistence of unscreened populations is at least part of the problem. Fifty percent of the women in the USA who develop invasive cervix cancer have not had a Pap smear in at least 5 years. Globally, carcinoma of the cervix represents a major public health priority, afflicting more than 400 000 women and causing more than 250 000 deaths annually.[2,3]

For many years, epidemiologic studies strongly suggested that cervix cancer has the features of a sexually transmitted disease (Table 6.1). In recent years, a causal relationship has been established between cervix cancer and infection with human papillomavirus (HPV). In studies of specimens obtained from 22 countries worldwide, Walboomers et al and

Table 6.1 Risk factors for cervix cancer.

- Infection with human papilloma virus
- No prior pap smear screening
- Young age at first coitus
- Multiple sex partners
- History of dysplasia, warts, or sexually transmited disease
- Smoking
- Age

Bosch et al demonstrated the presence of HPV in more than 98% of samples.[4,5] The exact mechanisms of carcinogenesis are still being elucidated, but it is clear that the interaction between the viral DNA and a host of cofactors launches a cascade of molecular events, which, if uninterrupted or not self-limited, transform cervix cells from a preinvasive to an invasive phenotype.[6] New and inexpensive tests for the presence of high-risk HPV sub-types are now available in the market and are likely to be incorporated into screening efforts in some way. There is a good chance that cervix cancer will be the first successful target of a vaccine for primary prevention of a malignancy.[7]

Although the incidence of cervix cancer has dropped since the introduction of the Pap smear, cervix cancer remains the leading cause of female cancer deaths in the world because of large unscreened populations. For a variety of reasons, Pap-smear screening is unlikely to succeed in societies with a weak medical infrastructure; therefore, multiple efforts are under way to develop quicker, more accurate screening technologies. Until these are perfected or a vaccine is introduced, cervix cancer will remain a worldwide women's health threat of a massive proportion.

Lymphatic mapping in gynecologic cancers has been pioneered in patients with vulvar cancer; however, the greatest impact of mapping may come in patients with cervix cancer. In this chapter, the rationale for lymphatic mapping in cervix cancer will be reviewed, as well as techniques and early results.

CLINICAL MANAGEMENT OF CERVIX CANCER

Contemporary management of cervix cancer begins with histologic confirmation of the diagnosis with directed biopsies. Diagnosis is followed by a limited radiographic survey and clinical examination, after which a stage is assigned, on the basis of which treatment decisions are made (Figure 6.1). A variety of imaging studies, including lymphangiography, computed tomography, magnetic resonance imaging, and positron emission tomography (PET), have been used in the evaluation of cervix cancer. The most recent and probably most sensitive method, PET, can detect metastases in the range of 7–8 mm.[8] Patients who have a target lymph node that can be imaged by computed tomography can safely undergo

O   Carcinoma in situ

I   Cervical carcinoma confined to uterus (extension to corpus should be disregarded)

IA   Invasive carcinoma, diagnosed only by microscopy. All macroscopically visible lesions—even with superficial invasion—are T1b/lb. Stromal invasion with a maximum depth of 5 mm measured from the base of the epithelium and horizontal spread of 7 mm or less. Vascular space involvement, venous or lymphatic, does not affect classification.

IA_1 Measured stromal invasion 3 mm or less and 7 mm or less in horizontal spread

IA_2 Measured stromal invasion more than 3 mm and not more than 5 mm with a horizontal spread of 7 mm or less

IB   Clearly visible lesion confined to the cervix or microscopic lesion greater than T1a2/IA_2

IB_1 Clearly visible lesion 4 cm or less in greatest dimension

IB_2 Clearly visible lesion more than 4 cm in greatest dimension

II   Cervical carcinoma invades beyond uterus, but not to pelvic wall or to the lower third of vagina

IIA   Tumor without parametrial invasion

IIB   Tumor with parametrial invasion

III   Cervical carcinoma extends to the pelvic wall and/or involves lower third of vagina or causes hydronephrosis or nonfunctioning kidney

IIIA   Tumor involves lower third of the vagina; no extension to pelvic wall

IIIB   Tumor extends to pelvic wall or causes hydronephrosis or nonfunctioning kidney

IVA   Tumor invades mucosa of bladder or rectum and/or extends beyond true pelvis

IVB   Distant metastasis

Figure 6.1   FIGO staging for cervical cancer.

percutaneous fine-needle aspiration prior to invasive surgical procedures to determine whether metastases are present.

Patients with advanced disease (stage IIB–IV) are almost always treated with a combination of teletherapy and brachytherapy. Recent evaluation of concomitant chemotherapy as a radiosensitizer suggests that its addition to the treatment protocol can be associated with prolonged progression-free and overall survival with acceptable augmentation of toxicity.[9–14] A recent meta-analysis of randomized trials of concomitant radiotherapy and chemotherapy by Green et al has confirmed reductions in the hazards of recurrence and death of 39% and 29%, respectively.[15] Efforts continue to identify the optimal radiosensitizing strategy in patients with advanced disease. Alternative management strategies for some of these patients (particularly those with stage IIB disease) involve a combination of three modalities, chemotherapy, surgery, and radiotherapy. Whether such strategies will ultimately improve overall survival will be resolved by ongoing prospective trials.

Surgery is generally reserved for patients in whom the primary tumor can be resected, intact with adequate lateral parametrial margins, and in whom the likelihood of metastatic spread is low. Cohorts of patients with stage IA2–IIA disease are often considered for radical hysterectomy as curative therapy. Candidate patients are usually younger, with good performance status, and interested in ovarian preservation. Patients whose vaginal/tumoral geometry precludes good brachytherapy application and patients in whom the likelihood of combined treatment (radical hysterectomy and radiotherapy) is low are also considered for radical hysterectomy. Recent studies have suggested that patients with smaller tumors (≤2 cm) may undergo type II radical hysterectomy without compromising their survival.[16–18] However, most patients offered surgery undergo type III radical hysterectomy with pelvic and low para-aortic nodal dissection. This procedure can be performed via laparotomy, laparoscopically, or vaginally (with laparoscopic lymphadenectomy). The incidence of unexpected metastatic nodal disease in these patients is less than 15–20% in most series, but it can be much higher in patients with stage IB2 and bulky IIA lesions.[18,19]

If positive lymph nodes are encountered in a patient with stage 1B1 or 1B2 cancer at the time of a planned radical hysterectomy, there is some debate over the best course of action. Some clinicians prefer to abandon the radical hysterectomy in favor of chemoradiation. There are several reasons for this approach. First, a high dose of radiation can be delivered to the primary tumor when the cervix is intact. Second, the local control rates with chemoradiation are outstanding.[20] Third, following radical hysterectomy and pelvic lymphadenectomy, there may be a higher risk of pelvic adhesions—in particular, adhesions of the small bowel to the vaginal cuff or pelvic sidewalls. This increases the risk of radiation enteritis if postoperative pelvic radiotherapy is given. Finally, radical surgery, along with chemotherapy and radiotherapy, is usually more expensive than chemoradiation alone.

Other clinicians prefer to complete the radical hysterectomy and pelvic lymphadenectomy even in the face of positive nodes. This strategy avoids the use of brachytherapy, which can result in high bladder and rectal doses, and the associated risks of radiation cystitis, proctitis, and even vesicovaginal and rectal-vaginal fistulas. These complications are very difficult to treat and usually necessitate a permanent colostomy or urinary conduit. In addition, there is some evidence that patients with only one microscopically positive node can be safely managed with surgery alone.[21]

Few randomized trials comparing the various treatment approaches in patients with stage IB1 have been conducted, but those completed show that the different approaches results in equivalent long-term survival.[19] A number of factors have been evaluated for their impact on prognosis, including age, race, socioeconomic status, anemia, chronic disease, HIV, tumor volume, local uterine extension, grade, and molecular profiles. The most important prognostic factor is lymphatic spread. Both number of involved nodes (1 vs ≥2) and location of involved nodes (pelvis vs, para-aortic vs both) appear to be prognostically significant.[22,23] Clinically, the pelvic chains are more frequently involved than the para-aortic nodes, and isolated involvement of the para-aortic nodes is uncommon (<3%).[24,25] However, morphologic characteristics of the primary tumor are not necessarily predictive of specific at-risk nodal reservoirs; as a result, complete lymphatic dissection (pelvic lymphadenectomy) or pelvic node irradiation is necessary for appropriate therapy.

It is very important for gynecologic oncologists to understand the preferences of the patient and the local resources in the medical community when making treatment decisions. For example, the Patterns of Care studies[26] consistently demonstrate that a large proportion of community-based radiation oncologists perform a very small number of brachytherapy insertions, and their complication rates are high. On the other hand, some hospitals might have poor critical-care facilities for patients undergoing radical hysterectomy who suffer severe surgical complications such as hemorrhage, embolism, or sepsis.

CERVIX CANCER AS A TARGET FOR LYMPHATIC MAPPING

Cervix cancer is an excellent target for the lymphatic mapping strategy (Table 6.2). Tumors are often detected early with Pap-smear screening or as a result of onset signs such as postcoital bleeding. The cervix is easily visible and accessible for injection both prior to and during surgery. The cervix is a midline structure with a complex drainage pattern. Treatment is based on the assumption of bilateral pelvic drainage; however, this basic assumption has never been investigated by in vivo techniques. The cervix has lymphatic drainage along several paths, as illustrated in (Figure 6.2). For this reason, regional lymphadenectomy requires extensive dissection. Even with an extensive regional lymphadenectomy, some nodal targets are not routinely removed, such as presacral and perirectal lymph nodes. Study of other disease sites has revealed how assumptions about in vivo anatomy can be incorrect. For example, Krag et al,[27] using preoperative lymphoscintigraphy, demonstrated that 6% of patients with early breast cancer have nonaxillary sentinel nodes, most commonly internal mammary nodes. Axillary lymphadenectomy misses the target sentinel nodes in these patients. Thompson et al[28] have shown how cutaneous lymphatic drainage pathways in patients with melanoma frequently do not conform to commonly accepted anatomic notions.

Lymph node status is the single most important prognostic factor in patients with cervix cancer. In patients undergoing radical hysterectomy and pelvic lymphadenectomy, survival drops by up to 50% when there are lymph node metastases, even with postoperative

Table 6.2 Cervix cancer as target for lymphatic mapping.

- Cervix is accessible to inject
- Midline structure with complex lymphatic drainage
- Lymph node status most important prognostic feature
- Lymph node status most important determinant for adjuvant treatment
- Sentinel node can be identified and removed laparoscopically

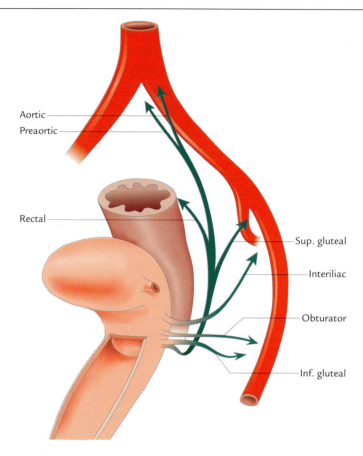

Aortic
Preaortic
Rectal
Sup. gluteal
Interiliac
Obturator
Inf. gluteal

Figure 6.2   The cervix is a midline structure with complex drainage. Plentl and Friedman described lateral collecting trunks with three branches, upper, middle, and lower. These trunks lead to lymph nodes in the iliac, common iliac, presacral, lower aortic, superior gluteal, and obturator locations. (Modified from Plentl and Friedman[33]).

radiotherapy.[12,19] The importance of accurate detection of positive lymph nodes is underscored by the recent success of chemoradiation trials. These studies[9–14] all demonstrated that chemoradiation significantly increases survival in node-positive patients compared with radiotherapy alone. Early detection of positive nodes will allow selection of chemoradiation prior to radical surgery where appropriate.

There is strong circumstantial evidence that lymph node metastases occur in an orderly fashion in patients with cervix cancer. For example, 5–6% of patients with stage 1B disease have positive aortic lymph,[30] whereas 15–20% have positive pelvic lymph nodes. This strongly suggests that common iliac or para-aortic lymph node metastases occur only in patients who have pelvic lymph node metastases. This forms the basis of the regional approach to lymph node treatment with both surgery and radiotherapy. Nevertheless, there may be a small number of patients with metastases to common, iliac, presacral, or para-aortic lymph nodes who do not have pelvic lymph node metastases.

The pelvic lymph nodes, including sentinel nodes, are accessible by several surgical techniques. These include transperitonel, retroperitoneal, and laparoscopic approaches.

Transperitoneal lymphadenectomy is the most common type combined with radical hysterectomy. If positive lymph nodes are encountered with this technique, surgeons have the option of continuing with radical hysterectomy or discontinuing in favor of chemoradiation with the cervix intact. The retroperitoneal approach allows for removal of lymph nodes without entry into the peritoneal cavity. This reduces the risk of adhesion formation and late radiation complications such as radiation enteritis. The most intriguing approach is laparoscopic sentinel node biopsy. This approach combines two less invasive techniques—laparoscopy and sentinel node biopsy—to determine lymph nodes status.

Patients with early disease—stage IA1 with lymph-vascular space involvement, stage IA2, or stage IB1—are the best candidates for lymphatic mapping and sentinel node identification. Patients with advanced cervix cancer are not good candidates for lymphatic mapping. Advanced tumors completely replace the cervix; therefore, there is no normal adjacent tissue into which to inject the blue dye (and sometimes radiocolloid) used in the mapping. In addition, patients with advanced disease are more likely to have altered lymphatic flow due to lymph nodes congested with tumor or inflammatory debris. In addition to advanced disease, other factors can interfere with the cervix as a target for lymphatic mapping. First and foremost, the tumor can be very close to the sentinel nodes. In this situation, lymphoscintigraphy may not be able to distinguish a sentinel node from high background counts at the site of injection of radiocolloid near the primary tumor. Medial parametrial nodes are not seen during a radical hysterectomy, and trying to find them could compromise the radicality of the operation.

LYMPHATIC MAPPING TECHNIQUE OF THE CERVIX

Sentinel node localization studies can be performed using vital blue dye, lymphoscintigraphy, or the combination. In the authors' experience, the combination technique is more robust and offers investigators with little experience performing lymphatic mapping the optimal opportunity to identify sentinel nodes in the large number of basins where they may be located. However, success during laparotomy and laparoscopy has also been reported with each individual agent used alone.

Preoperative lymphoscintigraphy

When lymphatic mapping is performed with a combination of vital blue dye and lymphoscintigraphy, the investigation begins with preoperative lymphoscintigraphy. This is performed in the nuclear medicine suite either the day before surgery or the morning of surgery. Approximately 1–1.5 ml of filtered ^{99m}Tc radiocolloid is injected with a 25-gauge needle into four quadrants around the cervical tumor. Steady pressure is applied through the needle to prevent spillage into the vagina. Thirty minutes after the injection, dynamic lymphoscintigraphy is performed with the use of a gamma camera (Figure 6.3).

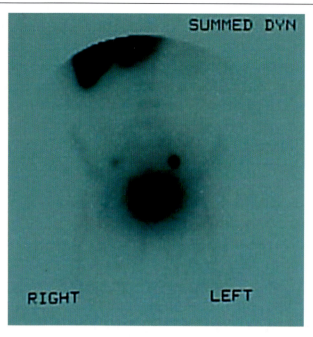

Figure 6.3 Approximately 1–.5 ml of filtered ^{99m}Tc radiocolloid is injected with a 25-gauge needle into four quadrants around the cervical tumor. Steady pressure is applied through the needle to prevent spillage into the vagina. Thirty minutes after the injection, dynamic lymphoscintigraphy is performed with the use of a gamma camera.

If lymphoscintigraphy is performed the day before surgery, static images are taken right before the patient is brought to the operating room. If lymphoscintigraphy is done on the day of surgery, static images are repeated for up to 180 min to identify at-risk nodes. Anterior–posterior and lateral views are obtained, with markers placed on bony landmarks such as the pubic symphysis and the anterior superior iliac crests. Since the half-life of the ^{99m}Tc used is approximately 6 h, patients in whom the radiocolloid is injected more than 18 h before surgery are given a second injection 1–6 h before surgery.

Intraoperative lymphatic mapping

On the day of surgery, following induction of anesthesia, the patient is placed in a low lithotomy position, allowing access to the cervix and facilitating abdominal incision (if laparotomy will be performed) or port placement (if laparoscopy will be performed). The cervix is then injected with vital blue dye (Figure 6.4). In the USA, the most commonly used dye is isosulfan blue 1% (Lymphazurin 1%, US Surgical Co., Norwalk, CT, USA). However, other investigators have reported success with patent V blue dye and with dilute (50:50) methylene blue dye (K. Fujiwara, personal communication). In the case of laparotomy, it is suggested that the laparotomy incision be performed prior to cervical injection of blue dye, given the very rapid uptake of dye and the short duration of nodal staining (median,

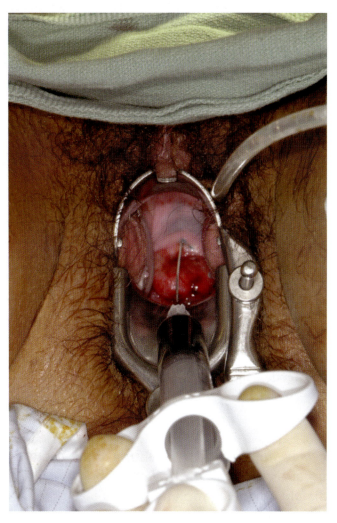

Figure 6.4 Injection of blue dye into the submucosa of the anterior lip of the cervix. The dye can be seen diffusing through the superficial lymphatics.

7 min). Dargent and colleagues have reported success with patent V blue dye alone in patients undergoing laparoscopy. In their experience, nodes stay blue for a much longer time (median, 20 min).[31] This may be due to the intra-abdominal pressures maintained by CO_2 gas insufflation. Regardless of the surgical approach—laparotomy or laparoscopy—3–5 ml of vital dye divided into equal portions is injected at four locations around the tumor 5–10 mm into the stroma. Immediately upon injection, there is blue staining of the parametrial tissues and bladder peritoneum. The retroperitoneum is carefully opened to permit visualization of the nodal basins and blue nodes. Intraoperative evaluation with a hand-held or laparoscopic gamma probe is performed to isolate and identify sentinel nodes (Figure 6.5). Both the pelvic and para-aortic regions are surveyed. The probe is collimated and angled laterally as much as possible to reduce the detection of residual radioactivity from the primary cervical tumor. Having the preoperative lymphoscintigram available in the operating room is helpful in the search for sentinel nodes. Close observation of the blue

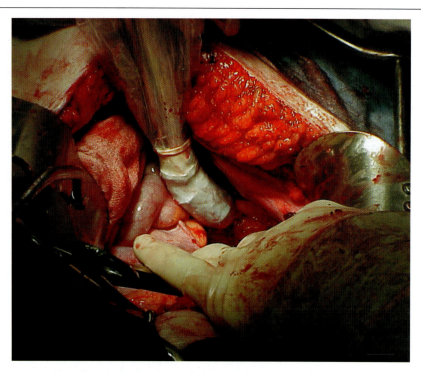

Figure 6.5 Interoperative use of the gamma probe to identify sentinel lymph nodes during radical hysterectomy. Note the probe is directed towards the pelvic sidewall and away from the cervix to aid detection of the sentinel lymph node which is less radioactive than the cervix.

lymphatic channels in the pelvis provides an insight into lymphatic anatomy of the pelvis and confirms the classic description by Leveuf and Godard[32] and Plentl and Friedman.[33] The most immediately obvious lymphatic channels are the lateral trunks (Figure 6.6). These trunks emerge from the cervix where the uterine vessels cross over the ureter. They traverse the loose areolar tissue that starts to form the web between the paraverical and pararectal spaces towards the pelvic vessels. A sentinel node is usually found at an interiliac or external iliac location.

The posterior trunks (Figure 6.7) are more difficult to find and trace. They are found deep in the pelvis in the loose areolar tissue of the pararectal space. They are finer than the lateral trunks and therefore contain less blue dye. If search for these trunks is delayed, the blue dye may be eliminated altogether. The posterior trunks will lead to a presacral sentinel node (Figure 6.8). These are usually smaller than the sentinel nodes lower in the pelvis.

Nodes retaining blue dye and nodes with gamma counts at least four times the background count are considered 'sentinel'. The 4:1 gamma-count ratio is used because, owing to the high circulating blood volume within the pelvis, background radioactivity can be registered in most locations. In our preliminary work using a combined technique, approximately 50% of sentinel nodes were both blue and highly readioactive.[34] However, approximately 25% of sentinel nodes were only blue and approximately 25% were only radioactive. Resection and gamma-count ratios above 10:1 ex vivo confirm sentinel node identification.

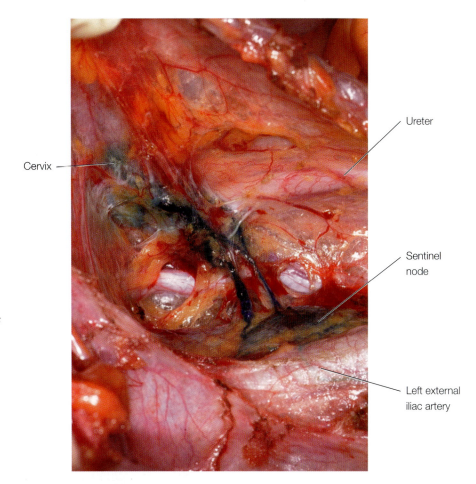

Figure 6.6 The upper branches of the lateral lymphatic trunks are seen originating from the left side of the cervix which is in the left upper corner of the photograph. They pass over the left ureter and terminate in a left interiliac sentinel lymph node. The left external iliac artery is at the bottom of the photograph.

Clinical experience with lymphatic mapping for cervical cancer and review of published trials

Clinical trials exploring the sentinel node concept in cervix cancer have been a very recent event. Table 6.3 summarizes the published trials to date of cervix cancer sentinel node mapping. The experience, although mixed in early trials, has generally supported the hypothesis that an identifiable, preferred lymphatic pathway from the primary tumor to its regional nodal basin exists. However, mapping in this disease site faces special challenges related to the tumoral injection, the high vascularity of the uterus, and the large number of pelvic and para-aortic lymphatic basins in which sentinel nodes may be found.

Blue-dye-alone experience

Echt and colleagues of the Moffitt Cancer Center were the first to report an experience with sentinel node identification among cervix cancer.[35] In this 1999 series, 13 patients underwent peritumoral injection of Lymphazurin 1% blue dye followed by laparotomy. In 12 of 13 patients, radical hysterectomy was completed; in one patient, hysterectomy was aborted following identification of a metastatic para-aortic node. Overall, just two (15%) of 13

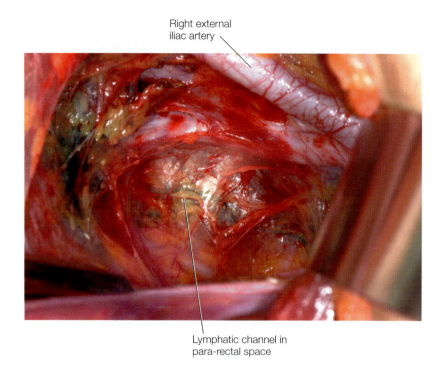

Right external
iliac artery

Lymphatic channel in
para-rectal space

Figure 6.7 Right lower branches of the lateral lymphatic trunk are seen in the pararectal space. These trunks originate from the cervix (or the left of the figure not seen) and usually terminate in presacral sentinel lymph nodes (behind the retractor on the right of the figure).

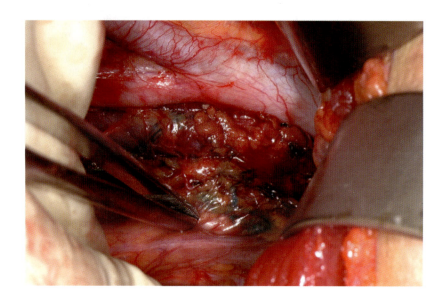

Figure 6.8 The same patient as figure 6.7 with further dissection demonstrating the right common iliac artery and the lymphatic channels terminating in small blue presacral sentinel lymph nodes. The pick up is resting on bone.

patients were found to have blue-stained sentinel nodes. In these two patients, both the blue sentinel nodes and unstained, nonsentinel nodes were found to contain metastatic disease. The patient with metastatic paraaortic disease (a solitary node) and the remaining 10 patients did not have an identifiable sentinel node. It is noteworthy that in this series just 2 ml of dye was injected and that these patients underwent injection before laparotomy. The authors concluded that modification of their technique would be required to permit future studies to assess accurately the sentinel lymph node concept.

Table 6.3 Published studies of lymphatic mapping and sentinel node identification in patients with cervical cancer.

Reference	Stage	Mapping Technique	Surgical Technique	Technical Success (patients)	False (−) (patients)	NPV	Sensitivity	SN Only (+) node
Echt, 1999[35]	IA-Ib	Blue dye	Laparotomy	2/13	0/2	0/0	2/2	1/2
Mendl, 2000[36]	Ib-IIA	Blue dye	Laparotomy	3/3	0/3	0/0	3/3	2/3
Verheijen, 2000[39]	Ib	Blue dye LS	Laparotomy	8/10	0/1	7/7	1/1	1/1
O'boyle, 2000[37]	Ib-IIA	Blue dye	Laparotomy	12/20	0/3	9/9	3/3	2/3
Dargent, 2000[31]	Ib	Blue dye	Laparoscopy	25/35	0/8	17/17	8/8	Unknown
Lantzsch, 2000[40]	Ib	LS	Laparotomy	13/14	0/1	12/12	1/1	0/1
Malur, 2001[43]	I-IV	Blue dye LS	Laparoscopy	39/50	1/6	33/34	5/6	Unknown
Levenback, 2002[34]	Ib	Blue dye LS	Laparotomy	39/39	1/8	31/32	7/8	6/8
Rob, 2002[38]	Ia-Ib2	Blue dye	Laparascopy Laparotomy	50/65	0	Unknown	Unknown	Unknown
Rhim, 2002*[53]	Ib	Blue dye LS	Laparotomy	25/26	1/5	20/21	4/5	Unknown
Barranger, 2002[44]	Ib	Blue dye LS	Laparoscopy	9/10	0/0	9/9	0/0	0/0
Plante, 2003**[45]	Ib	Blue dye LS	Laparoscopy Laparotomy	61/70	3/11	50/53	8/11	3/11
Marchiole, 2004***[46]	Ia-Ib	Blue dye	Laparoscopy	29/29	3/8	21/24	5/11	2/3
Total				315/384 (82)	9/56 (16.1)	209/218 (95.9)	47/59 (80)	17/32 (53.1)

Technical success: number of patients in which SLNs were found at surgery/total number of patients.
Sensitivity: proportion of patients with pelvic metastases in whom the SLNs contained tumor (true positive/[true positive + false negative]).
Negative predictive value (NPV): proportion of patients without tumor in SLNs in whom the pelvis was free of tumor (true negative/[true negative + false negative]).
Accuracy: proportion of patients with successful SLN biopsy in whom the status of the SLN correlated with the status of the pelvis ([true positive] + true negative/[true positive + true negative + false positive + false negative]).
LS, lymphoscintigraphy; SN, Sentinel node.
* Analysis of frozen section results.
** False-negative rate calculated by lmph node basin 0%.
*** Analysis based on scrial sectioning and immunohistochemistry of sentinel and non-sentinel nodes.

In a similar report, Medl and colleagues reported on three patients in whom the authors identified metastatic nodal disease using blue dye alone.[36] These patients had stage IB–IIA disease and underwent laparotomy following dye injection. In this trial, dye was injected into the lateral vaginal fornices rather than the cervical stroma. Although the authors expressed support for the adoption of sentinel node mapping for cervix cancer, they did not report the total number of patients studied, or whether there were any false-negative determinations.

Technical and clinicopathologic features influencing the success of sentinel node mapping were studied in a pilot project from the University of Texas Southwestern Medical Center in 2000.[37] The authors reported sentinel node identification in 12 (60%) of 20 patients undergoing laparotomy for early-stage (stage IB_1–IIA) cervix cancer. Tumor size (>4 cm) and prior conization were features associated with lack of sentinel node localization. The authors also commented that sequence might be important, given the rapidity with which blue dye is cleared from nodal tissues in the vascular pelvic basin. A total of 23 sentinel nodes were identified—15 in the interiliac and external iliac nodal chains, four in the common iliac basin, and four in parametrial tissues. Microscopic nodal metastases were found in four patients (20%), three of whom had disease in identified sentinel nodes. The fourth patient did not have an identifiable sentinel node. In addition, two of these four patients had bilateral nodal metastases, and in both patients only unilateral sentinel nodes (which were positive) were found. Nonetheless, for every sentinel node identified, the disease status of the node accurately reflected the disease status of the nodal basin.

Dargent and colleagues argued that lymphatic mapping and sentinel node biopsy would be most important for patients undergoing minimally invasive procedures, since validation of the sentinel node concept would limit the number of complete lymphadenectomies needed and pave the way for total vaginal resection or even fertility-sparing procedures, such as radical trachelectomy. In their series, 35 patients underwent laparoscopic mapping procedures and lymphadenectomy.[31] Defining 'success' as identification of a sentinel node on each pelvic sidewall, the authors reported that location (fornices vs stroma) and volume of dye (4 ml vs less) were significant predictors of a successful study. Overall, the authors identified sentinel nodes in 59 (86%) of 69 dissected pelvic sidewalls. In 51 instances, only a single dyed node was found on the sidewall. Interestingly, the median time between injection of dye and identification of a blue-dyed node was 52 min (range, 20–150 min). It is tempting to speculate that intra-abdominal pressure during laparoscopic procedures slows the clearance of dye. Metastatic disease was seen in 11 nodes (all sentinel nodes) from six patients. No false-negative studies were reported, although one patient had a metastatic node in a basin in which no sentinel node was identified. Details of sentinel node location in this study confirmed the importance of the lateral lymphatic trunks in cervical drainage. The interiliac, obturator, and external iliac basins (the so-called Leveuf et Godard area) were the location of 53 sentinel nodes.

Recently, Rob and colleagues presented their experience with patent blue dye lymphatic mapping in 65 patients undergoing laparoscopy ($n = 12$) or laparotomy ($n = 53$) for early cervix cancer.[38] Unique in this trial was the inclusion of 20 patients undergoing radical hysterectomy following neoadjuvant chemotherapy. Metastatic disease was found in three patients in the laparoscopy cohort, in all three cases within identified nodes sent for intraoperative frozen-section evaluation. There were no false-negative studies. The authors concluded that lymphatic mapping was feasible in smaller tumors with both laparoscopy and laparotomy, but was of limited use in patients with larger tumors following neoadjuvant chemotherapy. The authors further emphasized the importance of injecting the dye after port placement or laparotomy incision.

Lymphoscintigraphy experience

In an attempt to improve sentinel node identification and reduce the learning curve for lymphatic mapping procedures, many investigators have turned to lymphoscintigraphy, either as the sole technique for sentinel node identification or as an adjunct to the use of blue dye. Recently, Verheijen and colleagues reported their experience with radiocolloid mapping in 10 women with cervix cancer.[39] Focal uptake ('hot' nodes) was seen in six of 10 patients. Blue dye injection was also used in this study. Blue-stained nodes were found in four patients, and in all cases the blue-stained nodes were the same as nodes previously identified as 'hot.' A total of 18 sentinel nodes were detected at laparotomy, including in the single patient with metastatic disease. Most sentinel nodes were located in the external and interiliac chains, but sentinel nodes were seen in the common iliac basin in three patients. Bilateral sentinel nodes were seen in four patients.

Lantzsch et al detailed their experience with sentinel node identification using preoperative and intraoperative lymphoscintigraphy alone in 14 patients with stage IB disease.[40] This group performed intraoperative localization with a hand-held gamma probe and then completed radical hysterectomy and pelvic lymph node dissection. Focal uptake of filtered radiocolloid was seen in 13 patients (93%), and 26 sentinel nodes were identified. Five patients had bilateral sentinel nodes and eight patients had one or more unilateral sentinel nodes retrieved. One patient had histologically positive sentinel nodes. There were no false-negative studies.

A larger, multi-institutional experience was published by Levenback and colleagues, who used the combined blue dye–lymphoscintigraphy technique at laparotomy.[34] In this series, 39 patients underwent either preoperative ($n = 23$) or perioperative ($n = 16$) cervical stromal injection of radiocolloid. Localized uptake was seen on the lymphoscintigrams in 33 patients. All patients had at least one sentinel node identified, and bilateral sentinel nodes were found in 37 of 39 patients. Sentinel nodes in this trial retained either or both characteristics of blue and hot. Furthermore, size and preoperative cervical conization did not negatively affect identification of a sentinel node. Metastatic disease was found in 25 nodes from eight patients (Figure 6.9). In seven of these patients, at least one positive sentinel node was retrieved; in five, the only positive node was the sentinel node. In one patient with negative bilateral sentinel nodes, a positive parametrial node was identified in the hysterectomy specimen. The authors concluded that the addition of lymphoscintigraphy to the use of blue dye significantly improved their sentinel node identification rate and

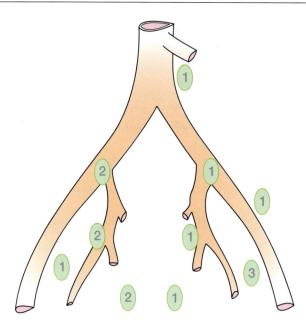

Figure 6.9   Green ovals show location of sentinel lymph node metastates in patients undergoing lymphatic mapping at time of radical hysterectomy.[34]

that more work in this area was needed to validate the technique. The identification of blue, not hot sentinel nodes in this trial needs further explanation and may relate to altered injection sites or clearance of radiocolloid with a short half-life. The relatively high radioactivity observed near the cervix following injection limits precise localization of nodes in the parametrium (unless the nodes are blue). The clinical relevance of these nodes with respect to survival has recently been called into question.[41]

Combined technique and laparoscopy

As was asserted by Dargent and colleagues, whose study is discussed earlier in this chapter,[31] laparoscopic sentinel node mapping may provide the greatest measure of benefit for patients with early-stage disease. There have been few published reports of use of a gamma probe with a laparoscopic approach, but the early reports support the feasibility of this technique and its importance in sentinel node localization.

In a letter to the editor, Kamprath and colleagues, presented data on 18 patients undergoing laparoscopic lymphadenectomy following preoperative radiocolloid injection.[42] Laparoscopic radical hysterectomy was performed in 15 patients, and radical trachelectomy was performed in three patients. Since no blue dye was used in this trial, resected nodes were secondarily scanned ex vivo for activity. Hot nodes were labeled sentinel and were found in 16 (89%) of 18 patients. Interestingly, a median of 2.1 pelvic sentinel nodes was found in the cohort, with a median of 1.4 para-aortic sentinel nodes being found among the five patients in whom such sentinel nodes were identified. The two nondiagnostic studies occurred in the first two patients in the series, who were given one-fifth and one-half, respectively, of the radiocolloid dose. One patient was found to have metastatic disease. This patient had one sentinel and three nonsentinel positive nodes.

Similarly, Malur and colleagues, from the same institution as Kamprath and colleagues, later reported their experience with patent blue dye alone ($n = 9$), radiocolloid alone ($n = 21$), and the combination ($n = 20$) in patients with early-stage cervix cancer undergoing pelvic and para-aortic lymphadenectomy via laparoscopy ($n = 45$) or laparotomy ($n = 5$).[43] The success and probability data from this trial by technique are presented in Table 6.4. The sentinel node detection rate was similar between laparotomy and laparoscopy (about 75%), although six patients in this series had stage IV disease and were undergoing extirpation by pelvic exenteration. Metastatic disease was documented in 10 patients (20%), six of whom had identifiable sentinel nodes. In all but one of these cases, the sentinel node contained metastatic disease. In two patients, the sentinel node was the only positive node. One patient with blue-dyed, histologically negative sentinel nodes was found to have a single positive nonsentinel node. This patient had lymphatic mapping with blue dye alone, prompting the authors to recommend the combined technique for further study. Among patients who underwent lymphatic mapping with the combined technique, 18 of 20 patients had sentinel nodes identified. Four patients had metastatic disease, and in all four cases, the sentinel nodes were positive.

In another letter to the editor, Barranger et al discussed their experience with laparoscopic sentinel node mapping following cervical injection of patent blue dye plus radiocolloid.[44] In this limited series of 10 patients, 1–3 sentinel nodes were identified in nine patients. No patients were found to have metastatic disease, but sentinel nodes were identified within the para-aortic region. The authors concluded that sentinel node mapping could have a role in minimally invasive surgical procedures for patients with early-stage cervix cancer.

Several recent studies using the combined technique demonstrate potential pitfalls with sentinel node biopsy in patients with cervical cancer. Plante et al[45] described a series of 70 patients mapped over a 2-year period as this group developed their expertise. During the initial phase of the study, the authors used blue dye only and used radiocolloid in the final 29 cases. There were no false negative sentinel nodes in the lymphatic basins studied; however, there were 3 patients with a negative sentinel node in one pelvic basin and a positive pelvic lymph node on the contralateral side. Sentinel nodes were not identified on the side with the positive node. Marchiole et al[46] successfully identified sentinel nodes in 29 patients

Table 6.4 Sentinel node blue/hot characteristics.

	Hot	Not hot	Total
Blue	65	35	100
Not blue	32	0	32
Total	97	35	132

primarily using blue dye. This group subjected all sentinel nodes to frozen section analysis. In addition, all sentinel and non-sentinel lymph nodes were subjected to serial sectioning and immunohistochemical staining for cytokeratins. There were 3 false negative cases. In each case, micrometastases were found in non-sentinel lymph nodes on immunohistochemistry only. This is the only study to subject all lymph nodes to ultrastaging. In other disease sites, frozen section of grossly normal sentinel nodes is avoided, since this process results in loss of tissue and degrades the quality of permanent sections. In addition, the authors bisected the sentinel node and did not obtain multiple sections ('bread loaf') as is generally recommended. The clinical significance of these micrometastases is uncertain.

TECHNICAL ISSUES IN LYMPHATIC MAPPING FOR CERVIX CANCER

Although it is controversial whether the combination of blue dye and lymphoscintigraphy offers an advantage over either modality alone, the combination approach most likely reduces the learning curve. Data from randomized trials of lymphatic mapping techniques at other tumor locations support this notion, with operator experience being the most significant factor.[47] In studies in which surgeons were allowed to use their preferred technique, no difference in sentinel node localization was observed between the modalities. However, the combined technique has been associated with a greater probability of multiple sentinel node identification, which has in turn been linked to a significant reduction in the rate of false-negative studies.[48] The development of a laparoscopic gamma probe has allowed combined-modality studies in patients undergoing laparoscopic lymphatic mapping. In all, fewer than 300 sentinel node-mapping procedures for cervix cancer have been documented; however, many clinical sites are testing feasibility and relevance.

Another clinical issue is that of rare allergic reactions to the blue dye agent—anaphylaxis, pseudoanaphylaxis, and 'blue hives'. This issue is discussed in detail elsewhere in the text, but is particularly pertinent to the mapping of the uterine cervix. Heightened vascularity of the cervix caused by carcinoma increases the likelihood of vascular uptake. We have previously reported a case of progressive arterial desaturation by pulse oximetry following cervical injection of Lymphazurin 1% dye.[49] This patient's well-being was confirmed by peripheral arterial blood gas determination, and it was suspected that 'competition' between dye pigment and dissolved hemoglobin measured by absorptive spectroscopy caused the incongruity. Nonetheless, anaphylactic reactions in 1–2% of patients have been reported with this and other dye agents.[29,50]

MOLECULAR BIOLOGY OF SENTINEL NODES IN CERVIX CANCER

Since much is already known about the pathogenesis of cervix cancer, examination of sentinel nodes may present an opportunity to learn more about the metastatic process in this disease model. Malur et al[43] have used molecular techniques to search for HPV DNA in pelvic lymph nodes. Although HPV DNA can be detected in the lymph nodes of women treated with radical hysterectomy, the significance of this finding is unclear. At least one investigator could not attach clinical significance to this finding in a small group of patients.[51] Van Trappen et al[51] have taken a somewhat different approach. They noted that a small number of relapses occur following radical hysterectomy and pelvic lymphadenectomy with all negative nodes. They hypothesized that histologically undetectable or dormant micrometastases were present at the time of lymphadenectomy. They used a highly sensitive reverse transcriptase polymerase chain reaction to detect cytokeratin-19, a marker expressed in epithelial cells, but not lymphoid cells. Cytokeratin-19 was elevated in the primary tumors of all 32 patients studied. Cytokeratin-19 was expressed in 66 (44%) of 150 histologically uninvolved lymph nodes and 16 (50%) of the 32 patients in the series. The highest levels of cytokeratin-19 were found in lymph nodes that correlate to the locations of sentinel nodes. Although Van Trappen et al did not perform lymphatic mapping, one could envision that sentinel nodes may in the near future be submitted for standard histologic analysis as well as molecular analysis. Much work will need to be performed to determine the clinical significance of 'biologic' metastases as described by Van Trappen and colleagues.

FUTURE DEVELOPMENT

Surgical validation of lymphatic mapping and sentinel node biopsy will require prospective investigation in more diverse cohorts, in a multi-institutional environment, and with adaptation of newer and more specific pathologic techniques, including molecular techniques, of nodal evaluation. Validation is required to support prospective, randomized trials in which individual treatment decisions are made on the basis of the sentinel node. Such trials are currently under development. It would seem that patients eligible for laparoscopic dissection would be ideal candidates for lymphatic mapping, as use of this technology would permit focal dissection and could permit fertility-sparing operations, such as radical trachelectomy.[52] In addition, sparing of potentially antigen-recognizing lymphoid cells could be critical to the successful adaptation of vaccine therapies for cervix cancer. Overall, however, more information about the clinical relationship between the primary tumor and its lymphatic basins is required to gain a deeper understanding of cervix cancer biology and unravel the mysteries of the clinical behavior of this disease.

REFERENCES

1. Hoskins W, Perez C, Young R. *Principles and Practice of Gynecologic Oncology* 3rd edn. (Lippincott Williams & Wilkins: Philadelphia, PA, 2000).
2. Jemal A, Thomas A, Murray T, et al. Cancer statistics, 2002. *Ca Cancer J Clin* 2002;**52**:23–47.

3. Janicek MF, Averette HE. Cervical cancer: prevention, diagnosis, and therapeutics. *Ca Cancer J Clin* 2001;**51**:92–114; quiz 115–18.

4. Walboomers JM, Jacobs MV, Manos MM, et al. Human papillomavirus is a necessary cause of invasive cervical cancer worldwide. *J Pathol* 1999;**189**:12–19.

5. Bosch FX, Manos MM, Munoz N, et al. Prevalence of human papillomavirus in cervical cancer: a worldwide perspective. International Biological Study on Cervical Cancer (IBSCC) Study Group. *J Natl Cancer Inst* 1995;**87**:796–802.

6. Park TW, Fujiwara H, Wright TC. Molecular biology of cervical cancer and its precursors. *Cancer* 1995;**76**:1902–13.

7. Koutsky LA, Ault KA, Wheeler CM, et al. A controlled trial of a human papillomavirus type 16 vaccine. *N Engl J Med* 2002;**347**:1645–51.

8. Grigsby P, Siegel B, Dehdashti F. Lymph node staging by position emission tomography in patients with carcinoma of the cervix. *J Clin Oncol* 2001;**19**:3745–9.

9. Morris M, Eifel PJ, Lu J, et al. Pelvic radiation with concurrent chemotherapy compared with pelvic and paraaortic radiation for high-risk cervical cancer. *N Engl J Med* 1999;**340**:1137–43.

10. Rose PG, Bundy BN, Watkins J, et al. Concurrent cisplatin-based chemotherapy and radiotherapy for locally advanced cervical cancer. *N Engl J Med* 1999;**340**:1144–53.

11. Whitney CW, Sause W, Bundy BN, et al. A randomized comparison of fluorouracil plus cisplatin versus hydroxyurea as an adjunct to radiation therapy in stages IIB–IVA carcinoma of the cervix with negative para-aortic lymph nodes: a Gynecologic Oncology Group and Southwest Oncology Group study. *J Clin Oncol* 1999;**17**:1339–48.

12. Keys HM, Bundy BN, Stehman FB, et al. Cisplatin, radiation, and adjuvant hysterectomy compared with radiation and adjuvant hysterectomy for bulky stage IB cervical carcinoma. *N Engl J Med* 1999;**340**:1154–61.

13. Pearcey R, Brundage M, Drouin P, et al. Phase III trial comparing radical radiotherapy with and without cisplatin chemotherapy in patients with advanced squamous cell cancer of the cervix. *J Clin Oncol* 2002;**20**:966–72.

14. Peters WA III, Liu PY, Barrett II RJ, et al. Concurrent chemotherapy and pelvic radiation therapy compared with pelvic radiation therapy aslone as adjuvant therapy after radical surgery in high-risk early-stage cancer of the cervix. *J Clin Oncol* 2000;**18**:1606–13.

15. Green JA, Kirwan JM, Tierney JF, et al. Survival and recurrence after concomitant chemotherapy and radiotherapy for cancer of the uterine cervix: a systematic review and meta-analysis. *Lancet* 2001;**358**(9284):781–6.

16. Landoni F, Maneo A, Cormio G, et al. Class II versus class III radical hysterectomy in stage IB-IIA cervical cancer: a prospective randomized study. *Gynecol Oncol* 2001;**80**:3–12.

17. Kinney WK, Hodge DO, Egorshin EV, et al. Identification of a low-risk subset of patients with stage IB invasive squamous cancer of the cervix possibly suited to less radical surgical treatment. *Gynecol Oncol* 1995;**57**:3–6.

18. Piver MS, Chung WS. Prognostic significance of cervical lesion size and pelvic node metastases in cervical carcinoma. *Obstet Gynecol* 1975;**46**:507–10.

19. Landoni F, Maneo A, Colombo A, et al. Randomised study of radical surgery versus radiotherapy for stage Ib–IIa cervical cancer. *Lancet* 1997;**350**:535–40.

20. Eifel PJ. Concurrent chemotherapy and radiation: a major advance for women with cervical cancer [editorial; comment]. *J Clin Oncol* 1999;**17**:1334–5.

21. Inoue T, Morita K. The prognostic significance of number of positive nodes in cervical carcinoma stages IB, IIA, and IIB. *Cancer* 1990;**65**:1923–7.

22. Tinga DJ, Timmer PR, Bouma J, et al. Prognostic significance of single versus multiple lymph node metastases in cervical carcinoma stage IB. *Gynecol Oncol* 1990;**39**:175–80.

23. Delgado G, Bundy BN, Zaino R, et al. Prospective surgical-pathological study of disease-free interval in patients with stage IB squamous cell carcinoma of the cervix: a Gynecologic Oncology Group study. *Gynecol Oncol* 1990;**38**:352–7.

24. Michel G, Morice P, Castaigne D, et al. Lymphatic spread in stage Ib and II cervical carcinoma: anatomy and surgical implications. *Obstet Gynecol* 1998;**91**:360–3.

25. Seski JC, Murray RA, Morley G. Microinvasive squamous carcinoma of the cervix. Definition, histologic analysis, late results of treatment. *Obst Gynecol* 1977;**50**:410–4.

26. Montana GS, Hanlon AL, Brickner TJ, et al. Carcinoma of the cervix: Patterns of Care Studies Review of 1978, 1983, 1988–89 surveys. *Int J Rad Oncol Biol Phys* 1995;**32**:1481–6.

27. Krag D, Weaver D, Ashikaga T, et al. The sentinel node in breast cancer, *N Engl J Med* 1998;**339**:941–6.

28. Thompson JF, Uren RF, Shaw HM, et al. Location of sentinel lymph nodes in patients with cutaneous melanoma: new insights into lymphatic anatomy. *J Am Coll Surg* 1999;**189**:195–204.

29. Dubost JL, Chevallier H. [Allergic reactions to patent blue violet: mechanisms, frequency and treatment]. *Phlebologie* 1982;**35**:739–46.

30. Lagasse LD, Creasman WT, Singleton HM, et al. Results and complications of operative staging in cervical cancer: experiences of the Gynecologic Oncology Group. *Gynecol Oncol* 1980;**9**:90–8.

31. Dargent D, Martin X, Mathevet P. Laparoscopic assessment of the sentinel lymph node in early stage cervical cancer. *Gynecol Oncol* 2000;**79**:411–15.

32. Leveuf J, Godard H. Les lymphatiques de l'utérus. *Rev Chir* 1923;**3**:219–48.

33. Plentl A, Friedman E. *Lymphatic System of the Female Genitalia* Vol. 2. (WB Saunders: Philadelphia, PA, 1971).

34. Levenback C, Coleman RL, Burke TW, et al. Lymphatic mapping and sentinel node identification in patients with cervix cancer undergoing radical hysterectomy and pelvic lymphadenectomy. *J Clin Oncol* 2002;**20**:688–93.

35. Echt M, Finan MA, Hoffman MS, et al. Detection of sentinel lymph nodes with Lymphazurin in cervical, uterine, and vulvar malignancies. *South Med J* 1999;**92**:204–8.

36. Medl M, Peters-Engl C, Schutz P, et al. First report of lymphatic mapping with isosulfan blue dye and sentinel node biopsy in cervical cancer. *Anticancer Res* 2000;**20**:1133–4.

37. O'Boyle JD, Coleman RL, Bernstein SG, et al. Intraoperative lymphatic mapping in cervix cancer patients undergoing radical hysterectomy: a pilot study. *Gynecol Oncol* 2000;**79**:238–43.

38. Rob L, Pluta M, Strnad P, et al. Sentinel node identification in uterine cervix cancer stage I: a pilot study. *Gynecol Oncol* 2002;**84**:521.

39. Verheijen R, Pijpers R, Van Diest PJ, et al. Sentinel node detection in cervical cancer. *Obstet Gynecol* 2000;**96**:135–8.

40. Lantzsch T, Wolters M, Grimm J, et al. Sentinel node procedure in Ib cervical cancer: a preliminary series. *Br J Cancer* 2001;**85**:791–4.

41. Winter R, Haas J, Reich O, et al. Parametrial spread of cervical cancer in patients with negative pelvic lymph nodes. *Gynecol Oncol* 2002;**84**:252–7.

42. Kamprath S, Possover M, Schneider A. Laparoscopic sentinel lymph node detection in patients with cervical cancer. *Am J Obstet Gynecol* 2000;**182**:1648.

43. Malur S, Krause N, Kohler C, et al. Sentinel lymph node detection in patients with cervical cancer. *Gynecol Oncol* 2001;**80**:254–7.

44. Barranger E, Grahek D, Cortez A, et al. Laparoscopic sentinel node procedure in patients with cervical cancer. *J Clin Oncol* 2002;**20**:2602; discussion 2602–3.

45. Plante M, Renaud MC, Tetu B, et al. Laparoscopic sentinel node mapping in early-stage cervical cancer. *Gynecol Oncol* 2003;**91**:494–503.

46. Marchiole P, Buenerd A, Scoazec JY, et al. Sentinel lymph node biopsy is not accurate in predicting lymph node status for patients with cervical carcinoma. *Cancer* 2004;**100**:2154–9.

47. Morrow M, Rademaker AW, Bethke KP, et al. Learning sentinel node biopsy: results of a prospective randomized trial of two techniques. *Surgery* 1999;**126**:714–20; discussion 720–2.

48. Wong SL, Edwards MJ, Chao C, et al. Sentinel lymph node biopsy for breast cancer: impact of the number of sentinel nodes removed on the false-negative rate. *J Am Coll Surg* 2001;**192**:684–9; discussion 689–91.

49. Coleman RL, Whitten CW, O'Boyle J, et al. Unexplained decrease in measured oxygen saturation by pulse oximetry following injection of Lymphazurin 1% (isosulfan blue) during a lymphatic mapping procedure. *J Surg Oncol* 1999;**70**:126–9.

50. Cimmino VM, Brown AC, Szocik JF, et al. Allergic reactions to isosulfan blue during sentinel node biopsy—a common event. *Surgery* 2001;**130**:439–42.

51. Van Trappen PO, Gyselman VG, Lowe DG, et al. Molecular quantification and mapping of lymph-node micrometastases in cervical cancer. *Lancet* 2001;**357**(9249):15–20.

52. Covens A, Shaw P, Murphy J, et al. Is radical trachelectomy a safe alternative to radical hysterectomy for patients with stage IA-B carcinoma of the cervix? *Cancer* 1999;**86**:2273–9.

53. Rhim CC, Park JS, Bae SN, et al. Sentinel node biopsy as an indicator for pelvic nodes dissection in early stage cervical cancer. *J Korean Med Sci* 2002;**17**:507–11.

7 SENTINEL LYMPH NODE MAPPING IN BREAST CANCER

Mary L. Gemignani

INTRODUCTION

Breast cancer remains the most common cancer in women in the USA. It is estimated that in the year 2004, there will be 215,990 new cases of breast cancer diagnosed in women.[1] The lifetime risk among women of developing breast cancer is 12.5% (1 in 8); the lifetime risk of dying from breast cancer is 3.6% (1 in 28). Although breast cancer remains a serious health concern in the USA, as well as in other countries, breast cancer mortality is declining in the USA and in other industrialized countries. This decline is thought to be secondary to the increased use of mammographic screening and early detection of breast cancer.

Axillary lymph node status remains the most important prognostic indicator in breast cancer. However, routine axillary lymph node dissection (ALND) in breast cancer patients often yields negative nodes, raising the question of unnecessary morbidity. Sentinel lymph node (SLN) biopsy in breast cancer evolved out of efforts to minimize the morbidity associated with ALND while still providing important staging information.

SLN mapping allows accurate surgical staging in patients with breast cancer. Successful identification of the SLN uses blue dye and/or radioisotope. Subsequent enhanced pathologic techniques provide increased detection of metastatic disease over conventional histopathologic methods.

BREAST CANCER

Natural history

Metastasis to the ipsilateral axilla is the most common route of spread. Metastasis to the internal mammary node is more likely in inner-quadrant lesions and is more likely to occur in the presence of axillary node involvement.

Pathology

Ductal carcinoma in situ

Ductal carcinoma in situ (DCIS) is classified as a heterogeneous group of lesions with distinct growth patterns and cytologic features. Classification is classically based on an architectural pattern and includes comedo, cribriform, and micropapillary patterns (Figure 7.1).

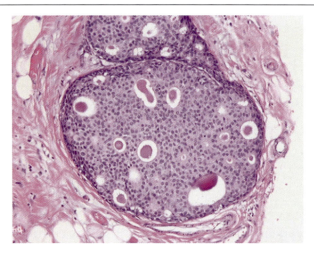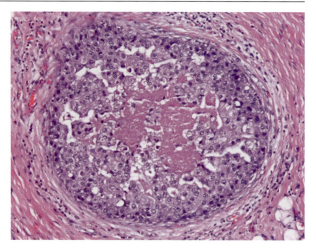

Figure 7.1 Ductal carcinoma in situ. A) Low-grade, ×100; B) High-grade, ×100.
(Reproduced with permission from Gemignani ML, Cancer of the breast. In: Editorial Committee (ACOG), *Precis: Oncology*, 2nd Edn, American College of Obstetricians and Gynecologists: Washington, DC, 2003, 17–33.)

Lobular carcinoma in situ

Lobular carcinoma in situ (LCIS) is a noninvasive lesion characterized by solid proliferation of small cells with round to oval nuclei distortion, the terminal duct-lobular units. It is not an invasive finding, but is thought to be a marker for increased breast cancer risk (Figure 7.2).

Invasive duct carcinoma

The category of invasive duct carcinoma comprises the majority of malignant mammary tumors (65–80%). Within this group are subtypes such as tubular, medullary, metaplastic, mucinous, papillary, and adenoid cystic carcinoma.

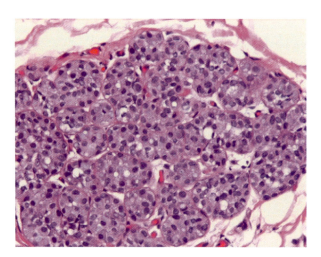

Figure 7.2 Lobular carcinoma in situ, ×200.
(Reproduced with permission from Gemignani ML, Cancer of the breast. In: Editorial Committee (ACOG), *Precis: Oncology*, 2nd Edn, American College of Obstetricians and Gynecologists: Washington, DC, 2003, 17–33.)

Infiltrating lobular carcinoma

Infiltrating lobular carcinomas constitute 10–14% of invasive breast carcinomas. These tumors tend to grow circumferentially around ducts and lobules, with a linear, 'India file' targetoid growth pattern.

STAGING FOR BREAST CANCER

The American Joint Committee on Cancer (AJCC) determines staging of breast cancer. The AJCC staging system is a clinical and pathologic staging system based on the tumor–node–metastasis (TNM) system. The new updated AJCC staging system (2002) incorporates sentinel node staging. It distinguishes micrometastasis from isolated tumor cells on the basis of size and histologic evidence of malignant activity. In the current AJCC staging system, supraclavicular lymph node metastasis is now classified as N3 disease, rather than M1 disease, as in the old system (Tables 7.1 and 7.2).

Table 7.1   American Joint Committee on Cancer Staging for Breast Cancer.

DEFINITION OF Tumor-Node-Metastasis (TNM)

Primary Tumor (T)

Definitions for classifying the primary tumor (T) are the same for clinical and for pathologic classification. If the measurement is made by physical examination, the examiner will use the major headings (T1, T2, or T3). If other measurements, such as mammographic or pathologic measurements, are used, the subsets of T1 can be used. Tumors should be measured to the nearest 0.1 cm increment.

TX	Primary tumor cannot be assessed
T0	No evidence of primary tumor
Tis	Carcinoma in situ
Tis (DCIS)	Ductal carcinoma in situ
Tis (LCIS)	Lobular carcinoma in situ
Tis (Paget's)	Paget's disease of the nipple with no tumor

Note: Paget's disease associated with a tumor is classified according to the size of the tumor.

T1	Tumor 2 cm or less in greatest dimension
T1mic	Microinvasion 0.1 cm or less in greatest dimension
T1a	Tumor more than 0.1 cm but not more than 0.5 cm in greatest dimension
T1b	Tumor more than 0.5 cm but not more than 1 cm in greatest dimension
T1c	Tumor more than 1 cm but not more than 2 cm in greatest dimension
T2	Tumor more than 2 cm but not more than 5 cm in greatest dimension
T3	Tumor more than 5 cm in greatest dimension
T4	Tumor of any size with direct extension to (a) chest wall or (b) skin, only as described below
T4a	Extension to chest wall, not including pectoralis muscle

T4b   Edema (including peau d'orange) or ulceration of the skin of the breast, or satellite skin nodules confined to the same breast

T4c   Both T4a and T4b

T4d   Inflammatory carcinoma

REGIONAL LYMPH NODES (N)

Clinical

NX   Regional lymph nodes cannot be assessed (e.g., previously removed)

N0   No regional lymph node metastasis

N1   Metastasis to movable ipsilateral axillary lymph node(s)

N2   Metastasis in ipsilateral axillary lymph nodes fixed or matted, or in clinically apparent* ipsilateral internal mammary nodes in the *absence* of clinically evident axillary lymph node metastasis

N2a   Metastasis in ipsilateral axillary lymph nodes fixed to one another (matted) or to other structures

N2b   Metastasis only in clinically apparent* ipsilateral internal mammary nodes and in the *absence* of clinically evident axillary lymph node metastasis

N3   Metastasis in ipsilateral infraclavicular lymph node(s) with or without axillary lymph node involvement, or in clinically apparent* ipsilateral internal mammary lymph node(s) and in the *presence* of clinically evident axillary lymph node metastasis; or metastasis in ipsilateral supraclavicular lymph node(s) with or without axillary or internal mammary lymph node involvement

N3a   Metastasis in ipsilateral infraclavicular lymph node(s)

N3b   Metastasis in ipsilateral internal mammary lymph node(s) and axillary lymph node(s)

N3c   Metastasis in ipsilateral supraclavicular lymph node(s)

* *Clinically apparent* is defined as detected by imaging studies (excluding lymphoscintigraphy) or by clinical examination or grossly visible pathologically.

Pathologic (pN)[a]

pNX Regional lymph nodes cannot be assessed (e.g., previously removed, or not removed for pathologic study)

pN0 No regional lymph node metastasis histologically, no additional examination for isolated tumor cells (ITC)

Note: Isolated tumor cells (ITC) are defined as single tumor cells or small cell clusters not greater than 0.2 mm, usually detected only by immunohistochemical (IHC) or molecular methods but which may be verified on HE stains. ITCs do not usually show evidence of malignant activity (e.g., proliferation or stromal reaction).

pN0(i −)   No regional lymph node metastasis histologically, negative IHC

pN0(i +)   No regional lymph node metastasis histologically, positive IHC, no IHC cluster greater than 0.2 mm

pN0(mol −) No regional lymph node metastasis histologically, negative molecular findings (RT-PCR)[b]

pN0(mol +) No regional lymph node metastasis histologically, positive molecular findings (RT-PCR)[b]

[a]Classification is based on axillary lymph node dissection with or without sentinel lymph node dissection. Classification based solely on sentinel lymph node dissection without subsequent axillary lymph node dissection is designated (sn) for 'sentinel node', e.g., pN0(i +) (sn).

[b]RT-PCR: reverse transcriptase/polymerase chain reaction.

pN1 Metastasis in 1–3 axillary lymph nodes, and/or internal mammary nodes with microscopic disease detected by sentinel lymph node dissection but not clinically apparent**

pN1mi Micrometastasis (greater than 0.2 mm, none greater than 2.0 mm)

pN1a Micrometastasis in 1–3 axillary lymph nodes

pN1b Metastasis in internal mammary nodes with microscopic disease detected by sentinel lymph node dissection but not clinically apparent**

pN1c Metastasis in 1–3 axillary lymph nodes and in internal mammary lymph nodes with microscopic disease detected by sentinel lymph node dissection but not clinically apparent** (If associated with greater than 3 positive axillary lymph nodes, the internal mammary nodes are classified as pN3b to reflect increased tumor burden)

pN2 Metastasis in 4–9 axillary lymph nodes, or in clinically apparent* internal mammary lymph nodes in the *absence* of axillary lymph node metastasis

pN2a Metastasis in 4–9 axillary lymph nodes (at least one tumor deposit greater than 2.0 mm)

pN2b Metastasis in clinically apparent* internal mammary lymph nodes in the *absence* of axillary lymph node metastasis

pN3 Metastasis in 10 or more axillary lymph nodes, or in infraclavicular lymph nodes, or in clinically apparent* ipsilateral internal mammary lymph nodes in the *presence* of 1 or more positive axillary lymph nodes; or in more than 3 axillary lymph nodes with clinically negative microscopic metastasis in internal mammary lymph nodes; or in ipsilateral supraclavicular lymph nodes

pN3a Metastasis in 10 or more axillary lymph nodes (at least one tumor deposit greater than 2.0 mm), or metastasis to the infraclavicular lymph nodes

pN3b Metastasis in clinically apparent* ipsilateral internal mammary lymph nodes in the *presence* of 1 or more positive axillary lymph nodes; or in more than 3 axillary lymph nodes and in internal mammary lymph nodes with microscopic disease detected by sentinel lymph node dissection but not clinically apparent**

pN3c Metastasis in ipsilateral supraclavicular lymph nodes

Clinically apparent is defined as detected by imaging studies (excluding lymphoscintigraphy) or by clinical examination.

**Not clinically apparent* is defined as not detected by imaging studies (excluding lymphoscintigraphy) or by clinical examination.

Distant Metastasis (M)

MX Distant metastasis cannot be assessed

M0 No distant metastasis

M1 Distant metastasis

Table 7.2 Stage by tumor, node, metastasis (TNM).

Stage 0	Tis	N0	M0
Stage 1	T1*	N0	M0
Stage IIA	T0	N1	M0
	T1*	N1	M0
	T2	N0	M0
Stage IIB	T2	N1	M0
	T3	N0	M0
Stage IIIA	T0	N2	M0
	T1*	N2	M0
	T2	N2	M0
	T3	N1	M0
	T3	N2	M0
Stage IIIB	T4	N0	M0
	T4	N1	M0
	T4	N2	M0
Stage IIIC	Any T	N3	M0
Stage IV	Any T	Any N	M1

*T1 includes T1 with microinvasion
Stage designation may be changed if post-surgical imaging studies reveal the presence of distant metastases, provided that the studies are carried out within 4 months of diagnosis in the absence of disease progression, and provided that the patient has not received neoadjuvant therapy.

THE AXILLA

At the time of Halsted's radical mastectomy, complete ALND was routine. The status of the axilla remains the most important prognostic factor for breast cancer.

The axilla is a pyramidal space between the arm and thoracic wall. It contains the axillary vessels and their branches, the brachial plexus and its branches, and lymph nodes embedded in fatty tissue. The primary route of lymphatic drainage of the breast is through the ipsilateral axillary lymph nodes (Figure 7.3).

The use of ALND has, in the past, been demonstrated to decrease significantly local recurrence. It is thought that a decrease in local recurrence may correlate with a survival advantage. A complete levels 1 and 2 lymph node dissection provides excellent local control, and local recurrence after this procedure occurs in less than 1% of patients. Metastatic involvement of lymph nodes is thought to occur in a stepwise manner. Rosen[2] demonstrated the incidence of 'skip metastasis' (that is nodal disease present in level 3, but in neither level 1 nor level 2) to be less than 2%.

The morbidity associated with ALND is significant. About 10–15% of patients develop lymphedema. In addition, numbness, pain, and/or weakness are often sequelae of this procedure.

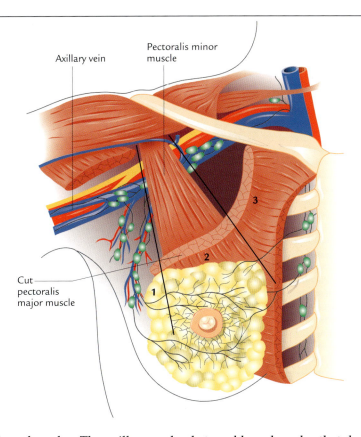

Axillary vein

Pectoralis minor muscle

Cut pectoralis major muscle

Figure 7.3 Axillary lymph nodes. The axillary and substernal lymph nodes that drain the breast are shown. The lymph nodes are also divided into levels by location relative to the pectoralis minor. Level 1 (low) lymph nodes lie lateral to the lateral border of the pectoralis minor muscle. Level 2 (mid) nodes lie behind the pectoralis minor muscle, and level 3 (high) nodes are medial (deep) to the medial border of this muscle. (Reproduced with permission from Gemignani ML, Sentinel lymph node mapping in breast cancer and melanoma, *Operative Techniques in Gynecologic Surgery* (2001)**6**:16–20.)

Prior to SLN biopsy, there was no adequate manner to address the status of the axillary lymph nodes without a lymphadenectomy. Clinical examination of the axilla is inaccurate, as often a negative clinical examination is not predictive of absence of metastatic disease. Multiple studies have shown that even in tumors less than 1 cm in size, lymph node metastasis may be present in more than 10% of patients. Other methods, such as axillary lymph node sampling (that is, removal of only a few random lymph nodes), are inadequate in predicting the extent of disease within the axilla compared with a standard ALND. The incidence of lymph node metastasis increases with larger tumor size.

SENTINEL LYMPH NODE (SLN) BIOPSY

The SLN concept was first introduced by Cabanas[3] in penile carcinoma. This concept proposed that the first lymph node in a regional lymphatic basin to receive lymph flow from a primary tumor, the 'sentinel node', would accurately reflect the status of the remainder of the nodes in that regional lymphatic basin (Figure 7.4).

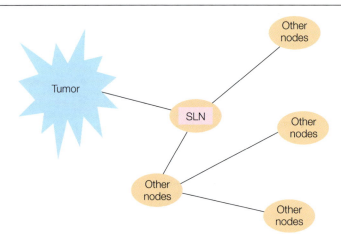

Figure 7.4 The sentinel lymph node (SLN) is the first lymph node that receives direct drainage from the primary tumor. Because it is the first site of drainage, it should be the first site of lymphatic spread. A tumor-free SLN implies the absence of lymph node metastasis in the entire lymphatic basin.

Initial studies in melanoma, by Morton and colleagues[4] in 1992, demonstrated the feasibility of the SLN concept in patients with cutaneous melanoma. This initial study of 237 patients used blue dye intradermally with successful identification of the SLN in 82% of patients. SLN mapping correctly predicted the regional nodal status in 99% of successful procedures and in 95% of node-positive cases.

Several studies have confirmed the accuracy of SLN biopsy.[5] In the majority of the studies, successful identification of the SLN occurs 92–98% of the time. The combination of blue dye and isotope has been reported to be better for identification of the SLN. The positive predictive value of the technique approaches 100%, with a negative predictive value close to 95% when both blue dye and radioisotope are used. The false-negative rate is about 5–10% in most studies (Table 7.3 [5–44]).

The validity of the SLN concept centers on the accurate predictability of the status of the regional lymphatic basin according to the SLN status. Turner [45] performed immunohistochemical (IHC) staining of all lymph nodes removed, sentinel and nonsentinel, in a series of patients undergoing standard ALND with clinically negative nodes. A total of 157 SLNs were examined; 10 (6%) demonstrated IHC positivity compared with only one of 1087 non-SLNs (0.09%). The authors concluded that the probability of non-SLNs containing metastases was less than 0.1% when both hematoxylin–eosin (HE) and IHC stains of the SLN were negative.

Axillary SLN biopsy with lymphatic mapping should be a consideration in the management of any patient with invasive breast cancer. SLN biopsy can be performed by a team that can proceed to ALND in the event that the SLN procedure is unsuccessful. It is not routinely indicated for DCIS and should be considered only if there is a suspicion of microinvasion. SLN mapping can be performed in conjunction with either mastectomy or breast-conservation therapy. However, in certain situations, a standard ALND should still be considered superior (that is, patients with clinically suspicious nodes). Contraindications for SLN biopsy with SLN mapping include pregnancy and patients with a suspected

Table 7.3 Validation studies of SLNB in breast cancer. (Adapted with permission from Liberman L, Cody HS III, Hill ADK, et al., Sentinel lymph node biopsy after percutaneous diagnosis of nonpalpable breast cancer, *Radiology* (1999) **211**: 835–44.)

Investigator/ year	Technical success rate	No. of SLN mean [range]	Sensitivity	Specificity	PPV	NPV	Accuracy	SLN is only site of disease (e)
Radioisotope series								
Krag/1993[6]	18/22 (82)	3.4 [NS]	7/7 (100)	11/11 (100)	7/7 (100)	11/11 (100)	18/18 (100)	3/7 (43)
Pijpers/1997[7]	30/37 (81)	NS [1–3]	11/11 (100)	19/19 (100)	11/11 (100)	19/19 (100)	30/30 (100)	7/11 (64)
Roumen/1997[8]	57/83 (69)	2 [1–4]	22/23 (96)	34/34 (100)	22/22 (100)	34/35 (97)	56/57 (98)	12/23 (52)
Galimberti/1998[9]	238/241 (99)	1.4 [1–4]	109/115 (95)	123/123 (100)	109/109 (100)	123/129 (95)	232/238 (97)	39/115 (34)
Borgstein/1998[10]	122/130 (94)	1.2 [1–3]	44/45 (98)	59/59 (100)	44/44 (100)	59/60 (98)	103/104 (99)[d]	26/45 (58)
Krag/1998[11]	119/157 (76)	3.0±2.0 [NS]	39/41 (95)	78/78 (100)	39/39 (100)	78/80 (98)	117/119 (98)	23/41 (56)
Offodile/1998[12]	40/41 (98)	3.0 [1–7]	18/18 (100)	22/22 (100)	18/18 (100)	22/22 (100)	40/40 (100)	NS
Crossin/1998[13]	42/50 (84)	2.0 [1–7]	7/8 (88)	34/34 (100)	7/7 (100)	34/35 (97)	41/42 (98)	NS
Krag/1998[5]	405/443 (91)	1.1 [1–3][a]	101/114 (89)	291/291 (100)	101/101 (100)	291/304 (96)	392/405 (97)	60/114 (53)
Snider/1998[14]	70/80 (88)	2.2 [1–5]	13/14 (93)	56/56 (100)	13/13 (100)	56/57 (98)	69/70 (99)	7/14 (50)
Miner/1998[15]	41/42 (98)	3 [NS]	7/8 (88)	33/33 (100)	7/7 (100)	33/34 (97)	40/41 (98)	4/8 (50)
Rubio/1998[16]	53/55 (96)	NS [1–4]	15/17 (88)	36/36 (100)	15/15 (100)	36/38 (95)	51/53 (96)	9/17 (53)
Gulec/1998[17]	30/32 (94)	2.5 [1–6]	8/8 (100)	22/22 (100)	8/8 (100)	22/22 (100)	30/30 (100)	5/8 (63)
Veronesi/1999[18]	371/376 (99)	1.4 [1–4]	168/180 (93)	191/191 (100)	168/168 (100)	191/203 (94)	359/371 (97)	70/180 (39)
Feldman/1999[19]	70/75 (93)	2.2 [±1.5]	17/21 (81)	49/49 (100)	17/17 (100)	49/53 (92)	66/70 (94)	7/21 (33)
Moffat/1999[20]	62/70 (89)	4.1±2.9 [1–12]	18/20 (90)	42/42 (100)	18/18 (100)	42/44 (95)	60/62 (97)	14/20 (70)
Subtotal	*1768/1934 (91)*	*1.7 [1–7]*	*604/650 (93)*	*1100/1100 (100)*	*604/604 (100)*	*1100/1146 (96)*	*1704/1750 (97)*	*286/624 (46)*
Blue-dye series								
Giuliano/1994[21]	114/174 (66)	1.7 [NS]	37/42 (88)	72/72 (100)	37/37 (100)	72/77 (94)	109/114 (96)	16/42 (38)
Giuliano/1997[22]	100/107 (93)	1.8 [1–8]	42/42 (100)	58/58 (100)	42/42 (100)	58/58 (100)	100/100 (100)	28/42 (67)
Guenther/1997[23]	103/145 (71)	1.6 [NS][b]	28/31 (90)	72/72 (100)	28/28 (100)	72/75 (96)	100/103 (97)	12/31 (39)
Flett/1998[24]	56/68 (82)	1.2 [NS]	15/18 (83)	38/38 (100)	15/15 (100)	38/41 (93)	53/56 (95)	5/18 (28)
Koller/1998[25]	96/98 (98)	2.7±1.2	48/51 (94)	45/45 (100)	48/48 (100)	45/48 (94)	93/96 (97)	13/51 (25)
Kapteijn/1998[26]	26/30 (87)	1.4 [1–3]	10/10 (100)	16/16 (100)	10/10 (100)	16/16 (100)	26/26 (100)	6/10 (60)
Imoto/1999[27]	65/88 (74)	2.0 [1–7]	25/29 (86)	36/36 (100)	25/25 (100)	36/40 (90)	61/65 (94)	9/29 (31)

Table 7.3 cont.

Investigator/year	Technical success rate	No. of SLN mean [range]	Sensitivity	Specificity	PPV	NPV	Accuracy	SLN is only site of disease (e)
Ratanawichitrasin/1998[28]	35/40 (88)	1.6±0.8	7/9 (78)	26/26 (100)	7/7 (100)	26/28 (93)	33/35 (94)	3/9 (33)
Dale/1998[29]	14/20 (66)	1.2 [NS]	5/5 (100)	9/9 (100)	5/5 (100)	9/9 (100)	14/14 (100)	3/5 (60)
Kern/1999[30]	39/40 (98)	2±1.5 [1–7]	15/15 (100)	24/24 (100)	15/15 (100)	24/24 (100)	39/39 (100)	7/15 (47)
Morgan/1999[31]	32/44 (73)	1.1 [1–2]	10/12 (83)	20/20 (100)	10/10 (100)	20/22 (91)	30/32 (94)	6/12 (50)
Morrow/1999[32]	110/139 (79)	1.8 [1–6]	28/32 (88)	78/78 (100)	28/28 (100)	78/82 (95)	106/110 (96)	12/32 (38)
Subtotal	*790/993 (80)*	*1.8 [1–8]*	*270/296 (91)*	*494/494 (100)*	*270/270 (100)*	*494/520 (95)*	*764/790 (97)*	*120/296 (41)*
Radioisotope + blue-dye series								
Albertini/1996[33]	57/62 (92)	2.2 [NS]	18/18 (100)	39/39 (100)	18/18 (100)	39/39 (100)	57/57 (100)	12/18 (67)
Borgstein/1997[34]	33/33 (100)	NS	14/14 (100)	11/11 (100)	14/14 (100)	11/11 (100)	25/25 (100)[f]	9/14 (64)
O'Hea/1998[35]	55/59 (93)	2.2 [1–8]	17/20 (85)	35/35 (100)	17/17 (100)	35/38 (92)	52/55 (95)	7/20 (35)
Barnwell/1998[36]	38/42 (90)	1 [1–3][c]	15/15 (100)	23/23 (100)	15/15 (100)	23/23 (100)	38/38 (100)	5/15 (33)
Nwariaku/1998[37]	96/119 (81)	1.8±0.9	26/27 (96)	69/69 (100)	26/26 (100)	69/70 (99)	95/96 (99)	18/27 (67)
Schneebaum/1998[38]	28/30 (93)	NS	11/13 (85)	15/15 (100)	11/11 (100)	15/17 (88)	26/28 (93)	1/13 (8)
Canavese/1998[39]	96/100 (96)	1.3 [NS]	28/33 (85)	63/63 (100)	28/28 (100)	63/68 (93)	91/96 (95)	8/23 (35)[f]
Czerniecki/1999[40]	41/43 (95)	2.6 [1–7]	15/15 (100)	26/26 (100)	15/15 (100)	26/26 (100)	41/41 (100)	7/15 (47)
van der Ent/1999[41]	70/70 (100)	2.6 [NS]	26/27 (96)	43/43 (100)	26/26 (100)	43/44 (98)	69/70 (99)	14/27 (52)
Bass/1999[42]	173/186 (93)	NS	53/54 (98)	119/119 (100)	53/53 (100)	119/120 (99)	172/173 (99)	NS
Burak/1999[43]	45/50 (90)	1.7 [1–5]	14/14 (100)	31/31 (100)	14/14 (100)	31/31 (100)	45/45 (100)	8/14 (57)
Jaderborg/1999[44]	64/79 (81)	1.9±1.2 [1–6]	19/20 (95)	44/44 (100)	19/19 (100)	44/45 (98)	63/64 (98)	14/20 (70)
Subtotal	*796/873 (91)*	*2.0 [1–8]*	*256/270 (95)*	*518/518 (100)*	*256/256 (100)*	*518/532 (97)*	*774/788 (98)*	*103/206 (50)*
Total	3354/3800 (88)	1.8 [1–8]	1130/1216 (93)	2112/2112 (100)	1130/1130 (100)	2111/2198 (96)	3242/3328 (97)	509/1126 (45)

SLN: sentinel lymph node; NS: not stated. Numbers in parentheses are percentages.

Technical success rate = proportion of patients in whom SLNs were found at surgery.

Sensitivity = proportion of patients with axillary metastases in whom the SLNs contain tumor (true positive / true positive + false negative).

Specificity = proportion of patients without axillary metastases in whom the SLNs are free of tumor (true negative / true negative + false positive).

Positive predictive value = proportion of patients with tumor in SLNs in whom the axilla contains tumor (true positive / true positive + false positive).

Negative predictive value = proportion of patients without tumor in SLNs in whom the axilla is free of tumor (true negative / true negative + false negative).

Accuracy = proportion of patients with successful SLNB in whom the status of the SLN correlated with the status of the axilla.

(true positive + true negative / true positive + true negative + false positive + true negative + false positive + false negative).

(a) Refers to number of hot spots (mean and range); an SLN was found underneath the hot spot in 405/413 (98%) women.

(b) Mean number of SLNs in women with histologically positive axillae. The mean number of SLNs in women with negative axillae was not reported.

(c) Median number of SLNs (mean not reported).

(d) Data refer to women who had successful SLNB and consented to undergo ALND.

(e) Indicates the proportion of women with axillary metastases in whom the SLNs were the only nodes containing tumor.

(f) Data for 73 clinically node-negative patients.

inadequate or aberrant drainage pattern such as may be caused by large tumors, multicentric tumors, or the presence of a large cavity produced from a prior excisional biopsy. For a patient with a previous large biopsy cavity that is near the axilla, caution should be used in relying on the SLN biopsy. This is due to the significant disruption of lymphatics that may have occurred from the prior excision. In general, however, larger tumors should not be considered absolute contraindications to the use of SLN biopsy if no clinically suspicious nodes are noted. Additionally, prior radiation therapy to the breast or neoadjuvant chemotherapy may alter the success/accuracy of SLN mapping. Proponents of continued complete ALND argue that the false-negative rate is too high to advocate the use of SLN biopsy in all breast cancer cases. It is likely that the false-negative rate will remain constant at 5–10%.

PATHOLOGIC ANALYSIS OF THE SLN

In contrast to conventional ALND, SLN biopsy has the advantage of facilitating the use of enhanced pathologic techniques, such as IHC, for the evaluation of the SLNs. Overall, greater scrutiny is paid to SLNs through serial sectioning and IHC staining. Serial sectioning improves the detection of metastases and increases the yield (up to 30%) in HE analysis over single sectioning[46,47] and, along with IHC staining, is possible in SLN biopsy because only a few SLNs are obtained at the time of the procedure. Neither serial sectioning nor IHC would be practical or cost-effective in a standard ALND, which yields an average of 20 nodes.

IHC stains used in breast cancer are monoclonal antibodies against the cytokeratins AE1/AE3 and CAM 5.2. Several studies have demonstrated an increase in the diagnostic yield of occult nodal metastases with the use of IHC analysis in patients thought to have negative nodes through standard histologic analysis using HE stains. Use of IHC stains can increase the yield of detection of tumor cells by 10–20% over standard histopathologic analysis. Metastases less than 2 mm in size are classified as micrometastases.[48] The clinical significance of micrometastases is currently debated; however, the Ludwig study[49] has shown that patients with micrometastases have a worse 5-year survival than those with no metastases, namely, true node-negative patients. The impact on overall survival may be altered as adjuvant therapy is altered by enhanced histopathologic techniques and detection of metastatic disease (Figure 7.5). SLN biopsy makes enhanced pathologic analysis logistically feasible and allows identification of a group of patients with increased risk of systematic relapse who might otherwise be unrecognized.

The issue of isolated micrometastatic disease in the SLN is an area of controversy. The question of whether everyone with a positive SLN needs a complete ALND is debatable. The accuracy, value, and future of SLN biopsy currently is being evaluated in several prospective national trials. Among these trials is the American College of Surgeons Oncology Group (ACOSOG) Z0010 and Z0011 trials.

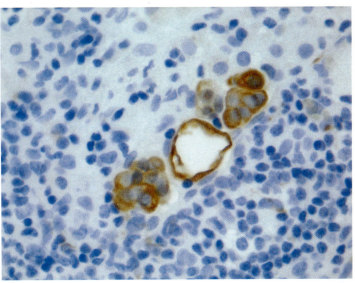

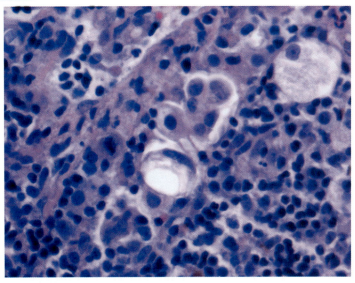

Figure 7.5 Metastases identified with immunohistochemical (IHC) stains in a patient who underwent SLN mapping. The use of ultrastaging techniques, such as IHC stains, will improve the rate of detection of lymph node metastasis over HE alone. Serial sectioning of resected nodes improves detection of occult metastases. Combination of serial sectioning and IHC stains will improve detection of metastatic disease in otherwise HE negative nodes.

The ACOSOG Z0011 trial randomly assigns women with clinical T1 or T2 N0M0 breast cancer and a positive SLN to one of two treatment arms: ALND or no ALND. The primary endpoint is overall survival. Secondary endpoints are surgical morbidities and disease-free survival. If no difference is seen, patients can potentially be spared the morbidity of an ALND, even in the positive SLN setting.

Until data are available, the standard of care for SLN-positive patients is ALND.

Supporters of the SCOSOG Z0011 trial cite the fact that the SLN is the only positive node in the majority of patients. With increasing mammographic screening, the size of primary breast cancers at diagnosis has shown a downward trend, thus being associated with a reduction in the number of tumor-positive axillary lymph nodes.[50]

Studies have shown that the SLN is the only site of nodal metastases in 40–60% of axillary node dissections.[5,21,33,35] In addition, the administration of adjuvant chemotherapy is not solely dependent on the axillary lymph node status, and the majority of patients receive adjuvant chemotherapy.

INTRAOPERATIVE TECHNIQUES

Frozen-section analysis allows visualization of the nodal architecture. It has been reported to have a false-negative rate of 6–24% compared with final analysis on paraffin.[46,47] Frozen-section analysis is more reliable for macrometastatic disease ([CLOSECHEV]2 mm). Disadvantages of this technique include frozen-tissue artifact, the consumption of tissue, and intraoperative delay.

The use of imprint cytology has also been reported in SLN mapping. Imprint cytology uses touch preparations, which can provide excellent cytologic detail and allow rapid analysis, as well as increased tissue preservation for use in paraffin sections. The inherent limitations of imprint cytology, however, are the smaller number of cells examined compared with frozen-section analysis, and the associated higher incidence of indeterminate results.

In breast cancer, intraoperative frozen-section analysis has the potential to alter surgical management: if metastases are noted in the SLN on frozen-section analysis, proceeding with an ALND is indicated. We reported on the charges associated with SLN procedures in 50 patients with T1 tumors at Memorial Hospital. We noted that although the intraoperative frozen-section analysis contributed significantly to the cost of the procedure, it identified eight patients (16%) with positive nodes who went on to have immediate ALND, in each case avoiding the need for a subsequent operation.[51] The value of the frozen section was in identifying a positive sentinel node and thus sparing the patient a reoperation.

TECHNICAL ISSUES: BLUE DYE AND ISOTOPE

Isosulfan blue dye (Lymphazurin, Hirsch Industries, Richmond, VA, USA) is a monosodium salt of a 2,5-disulfonated triphenyl methane dye.[52] It binds weakly to albumin and is taken up selectively by the lymphatics. It has a less than 1% incidence of allergic reactions. These include urticaria, rashes, and 'blue hives'. However, anaphylactic reactions with cardiovascular collapse have also been reported.

A recent report on the incidence of allergic reaction involving isosulfan blue dye at Memorial Sloan-Kettering Cancer Center reported the incidence of documented allergic reactions in 39 of 2392 patients (1.6%) undergoing SLN biopsy. The majority of the reactions (69%) were blue hives and urticaria. The incidence of hypotensive reaction was 0.5%. Bronchospasm and respiratory compromise were noted to be unusual events not requiring emergency intubation. Short-term pressor support was needed in these unusual events. There was no cross-sensitivity to sulfa allergy and isosulfan-blue-dye administration.[53]

Patent blue-V dye is a triphenyl methane dye similar to isosulfan blue that is used in Europe. Patent blue-V dye has been used in lymphangiography longer than isosulfan blue dye. The frequency of allergic reactions to patent blue dye has been estimated to be 0.2–2.7%.[54,55]

In 1982, isosulfan blue dye was approved by the Food and Drug Administration for lymphatic mapping. It is the only compound approved in the USA for SLN mapping.[52]

RADIOISOTOPE/NUCLEAR MEDICINE

In the USA, the majority of the published experience has been with technetium-99m ^{99m}Tc sulfur colloid (^{99m}Tc-SC), while in Europe, ^{99m}Tc colloidal albumin is used. Filtration of the colloid produces uniformity of particle size and is standard in lymphatic mapping in melanoma. In breast cancer, the unfiltered colloid has been reported to be more helpful in lymphatic mapping.[56]

Lymphoscintigraphy is an important component of SLN mapping in patients with melanoma, as it identifies anomalous patterns and correctly identifies the lymphatic basin to be investigated. This is less important in breast cancer, where the ipsilateral axilla is the primary focus. A negative lymphoscintigram does not preclude successful intraoperative localization of the SLN.

Radioisotope used in SLN biopsy succeeds more often than blue dye alone. A number of studies have found that SLN identified by intraparenchymal, subdermal, intradermal, or subareolar injection stage the axilla with comparable accuracy.

It is thought that the entire breast and overlying skin function as one, with drainage to an identifiable sentinel lymph node in most patients.[57] This may explain why such a wide variation in isotope techniques, including dosage, medium location, and timing of injection, produces a similarity in outcome for identification of the SLN.

THE LEARNING CURVE

A learning curve has been reported to be associated with the procedure.[58] The success at identifying the SLN is increased with a surgeon's increased experience.

The specific number of cases, complete with backup ALND, that are required is currently unresolved. It is recommended, however, that all SLN procedures done during the initial period of training be validated by backup ALND to determine the accuracy as well as the false-negative rate for the procedure during this initial period. In the literature, there are reports of the use of blue dye alone, radioisotope alone, and the two in combination. The use of blue dye and isotope together has been shown to increase the success of identifying the SLN and may help to decrease the associated learning curve for this procedure. It is also very important that an unsatisfactory intraoperative mapping be followed by an immediate ALND.

Bass et al[42] found that to identify the SLN, surgeons required an average of 23 cases to achieve 90% success and 53 cases to achieve 95% success, although the SLN was falsely negative in only 2% of their node-positive patients.

Most studies recommend that the first 20–30 SLN biopsy procedures be done with a backup ALND. McMasters et al,[59] however, reported in a multi-institutional trial that after 10 SLN operations, the frequency of successful mapping and false-negative results was similar among the many surgeons in the trial. Additionally, it was noted that false-negatives occur half as often with a combined technique as with a single-agent technique.

THE SLN MAPPING PROCEDURE

Our current approach at Memorial Sloan-Kettering Cancer Center is to use both isotope and blue-dye for lymphatic mapping.[60]

The morning of the operation, the patient receives 0.1 mCi of unfiltered ^{99m}Tc-SC (CIS-U.S. Inc., Bedford, MA, USA) intradermally overlying the site of the tumor. Alternatively the night before surgery, mapping is often employed. This has not been demonstrated to have a negative impact in successful SLN identification. A lymphoscintigram is obtained preoperatively (Figure 7.6).

One to two hours after the isotope injection, the patient is taken to the operating room. Under either local or general anesthesia, the breast and axilla are prepped and draped in the usual manner, and an intraparenchymal injection of 2–4 ml of isosulfan blue dye is injected close to the location of the tumor (Figures 7.7–7.11). Within 5–10 min, the axilla is explored through a small transverse incision (Figure 7.12). Identification and removal of all hot and blue nodes is done with the aid of the hand-held gamma probe and identification of the blue lymphatic channels (Figures 7.13–7.16).

The SLN(s) is submitted for frozen-section analysis, and if metastases are identified, an immediate ALND is performed. If the frozen section is negative, subsequent enhanced pathology is performed. If further studies, serial sectioning, and/or IHC stains reveal positive nodes, the patient is given the recommendation for ALND.

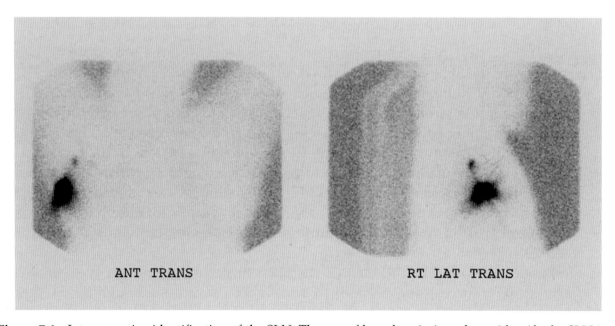

Figure 7.6 Intraoperative identification of the SLN. The use of lymphoscintigraphy to identify the SLN in melanoma is well documented. The value of the preoperative lymphoscintigram in SLN mapping in breast cancer is controversial. Injection of radioisotope in conjunction with blue dye has been shown to increase the success of finding the SLN and thus decrease the learning curve associated with the procedure.

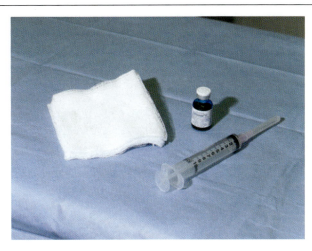

Figure 7.7 Injection of the blue dye at the time of surgery is helpful in the SLN procedure. Adverse reactions are around 1% and the use of the blue dye in conjunction with radioisotope increases the success rate of lymphatic mapping compared to either technique alone. The success with blue dye also remains low at about 60%.

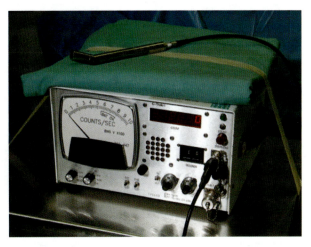

Figure 7.8 The gamma probe (C-Trak, Care Wise, Inc., Morgan Hill, CA, USA) can be used to identify intraoperatively the 'hot' SLN during dissection. The gamma probe provides an auditory signal that can help direct the dissection toward the location of the SLN.

It is important to perform careful intraoperative palpation of the axilla. Proceeding with the standard ALND in light of suspicious findings is important. Cody and colleagues[58,61] reported that in greater than 50% of false-negative SLN biopsy procedures, clinically suspicious nodes were present. In these cases, gross tumor involvement of the nodes may ultimately impair the uptake of both isotope and dye by the true sentinel node.

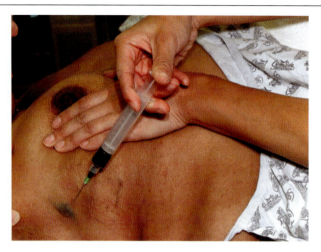

Figure 7.9 Injection of the blue dye can also be performed intradermally, but will require a smaller volume. It is important to note that large prior excisional cavities may decrease the success of the lymphatic mapping procedure, as disruption of the lymphatics may play a significant role in these cases.

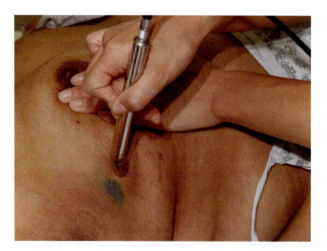

Figure 7.10 The radioactive counts help to determine the amount of radioisotope that is present in the injection site.

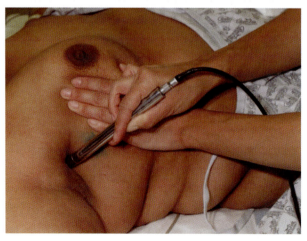

Figure 7.11 The area of maximum radioactivity is noted. Surgical exploration will begin directly over this area to have greatest potential in identification of the SLN.

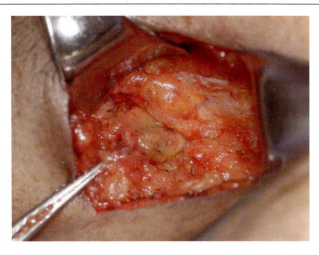

Figure 7.12   Careful dissection is performed so as not to disrupt the blue lymphatics, which will lead to the SLN.

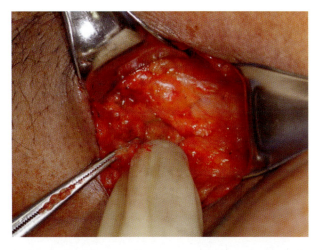

Figure 7.13   The gamma probe is dressed with a sterile cover and is used to help localize the direction to proceed for identification of the SLN.

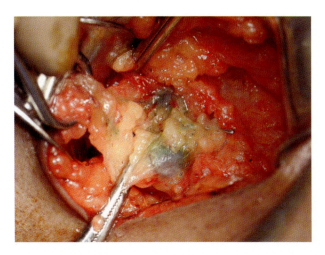

Figure 7.14   Identification of the 'blue' SLN is noted.

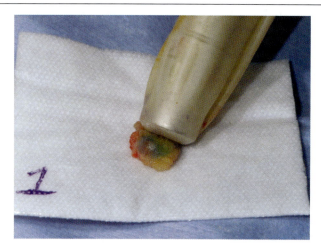

Figure 7.15   The use of both radioisotope and blue dye will ensure success for the SLN procedure. An average of two nodes is usually found during this procedure. However, any blue or hot node will need to be removed to decrease the rate of a false-negative procedure.

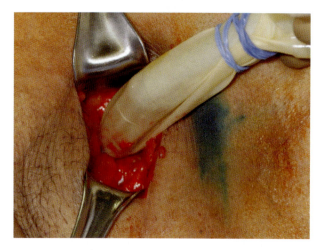

Figure 7.16   After removal of the blue nodes, the gamma probe is introduced into the axilla to check for any residual radioactivity hotspots, which may indicate an additional SLN. A fourfold decrease in counts is considered a successful radiolocalization. This reduced count is recorded.

FOLLOW-UP

Local recurrence after SLN biopsy for melanoma has been reported.[62] Recent reports have found that the rates of isolated axillary relapse after a negative SLN biopsy are comparable to a conventional ALND, namely, 1% or less. Chung et al[63] found three axillary recurrences in 206 patients with negative SLNs. Blanchard et al[64] found one axillary recurrence in 685 SLN negative women with 2-year follow-up.

The long-term morbidities of SLN biopsy will require long-term follow-up. A prospective trial looking at sensory morbidity after SLN biopsy and ALND found sensory deficits in the SLN group of one-half the magnitude of that found in patients undergoing ALND.[65] Lymphedema studies will require longer follow-up.

CONCLUSION

The SLN procedure allows improved staging in patients with breast cancer through greater scrutiny by enhanced histopathologic techniques and increased detection of metastases. This, in turn, may alter prognosis by altering adjuvant therapy. SLN mapping also affords decreased morbidity by avoiding regional lymphadenectomy in patients with breast cancer and negative SLNs.

REFERENCES

1. Jemal A, Murray T, Samuels A, et al. Cancer statistics, 2003. *CA Cancer J Clin* 2003;**53**:5–26.
2. Rosen PP. Discontinuous or 'skip' metastases in breast carcinoma. Analysis of 1228 axillary dissections. *Ann Surg* 1983;**197**:276–83.
3. Cabanas R. An approach for the treatment of penile carcinoma. *Cancer* 1977;**39**:456–66.
4. Morton DL. Technical details of intraoperative lymphatic mapping for early stage melanoma. *Arch Surg* 1992;**127**:392–9.
5. Krag D. The sentinel node in breast cancer—a multicenter validation study. *N Engl J Med* 1998;**339**:941–6.
6. Krag DN, Weaver DL, Alex JC, et al. Surgical resection and radiolocalization of the sentinel lymph node in breast cancer using a gamma probe. *Surg Oncol* 1993;**2**:335–40.
7. Pijpers R, Hoekstra OS, Collet GJ, et al. Impact of lymphoscintigraphy on sentinel node identification with technetium-99m-colloidal albumin in breast cancer. *J Nucl Med* 1997;**38**:366–8.
8. Roumen RMH, Valkenburg JGM, Geuskens LM. Lymphoscintigraphy and feasibility of sentinel node biopsy in 83 patients with primary breast cancer. *Eur J Surg Oncol* 1997;**23**:495–502.
9. Galimberti V, Zurrida S, Zucali P, et al. Can sentinel node biopsy avoid axillary dissection in clinically node-negative breast cancer patients? *Breast* 1998;**7**:8–10.
10. Borgstein PJ, Pijpers R, Comans EF, et al. Sentinel lymph node biopsy in breast cancer: guidelines and pitfalls of lymphoscintigraphy and gamma probe detection. *J Am Coll Surg* 1998;**186**:275–83.
11. Krag DN, Ashikaga T, Harlow SP, et al. Development of sentinel node targeting technique in breast cancer patients. *Breast J* 1998;**4**:67–74.
12. Offodile R, Hoh C, Barsky SH, et al. Minimally invasive breast carcinoma staging using lymphatic mapping with radiolabeled dextran. *Cancer* 1998;**82**:1704–8.
13. Crossin JA, Johnson AC, Stewart PB, et al. Gamma-probe-guided resection of the sentinel lymph node in breast cancer. *Am Surg* 1998;**64**:666–9.
14. Snider H, Dowlatshahi K, Fan M, et al. Sentinel node biopsy in the staging of breast cancer. *Am J Surg* 1998;**176**:305–10.

15. Miner TJ, Shriver CD, Jaques DP, et al. Ultrasonographically guided injection improves localization of the radiolabeled sentinel lymph node in breast cancer. *Ann Surg Oncol* 1998;**5**:315–21.

16. Rubio IT, Korourian S, Cowan C, et al. Sentinel lymph node biopsy for staging breast cancer. *Am J Surg* 1998;**176**:532–7.

17. Gulec SA, Moffat FL, Carroll RG, et al. Sentinel lymph node localization in early breast cancer. *J Nucl Med* 1998;**39**:1388–93.

18. Veronesi U, Paganelli G, Viale G, et al. Sentinel lymph node biopsy and axillary dissection in breast cancer: results in a large series. *J Natl Cancer Inst* 1999;**91**:368–73.

19. Feldman S, Krag DN, McNally RK, et al. Limitation in gamma probe localization of the sentinel node in breast cancer patients with large excisional biopsy. *J Am Coll Surg* 1999;**188**:248–54.

20. Moffat FL, Gulec SA, Sittler SY, et al. Unfiltered sulfur colloid and sentinel node biopsy for breast cancer: technical and kinetic considerations. *Ann Surg Oncol* 1999;**6**:746–55.

21. Giuliano AE, Kirgan DM, Guenther JM, et al. Lymphatic mapping and sentinel lymphadenectomy for breast cancer. *Ann Surg* 1994;**220**:391–401.

22. Giuliano AE, Jones RC, Brennan M, et al. Sentinel lymphadenectomy in breast cancer. *J Clin Oncol* 1997;**15**:2345–50.

23. Guenther JM, Krishnamoorthy M, Tan LR. Sentinel lymphadenectomy for breast cancer in a community managed care setting. *Cancer J Sci Am* 1997;**3**:336–40.

24. Flett MM, Going JJ, Stanton PD, et al. Sentinel node localization in patients with breast cancer. *Br J Surg* 1998;**85**:991–3.

25. Koller M, Barsuk D, Zippel D, et al. Sentinel lymph node involvement—a predictor for axillary node status with breast cancer—has the time come? *Eur J Surg Oncol* 1998;**24**:166–8.

26. Kapteijn BAE, Nieweg OE, Petersen JL, et al. Identification and biopsy of the sentinel lymph node in breast cancer. *Eur J Surg Oncol* 1998;**24**:427–30.

27. Imoto S, Hasebe T. Initial experience with sentinel node biopsy in breast cancer at the National Cancer Center Hospital East. *Jpn J Clin Oncol* 1999;**29**:11–15.

28. Ratanawichitrasin A, Levy L, Myles J, et al. Experience with lymphatic mapping in breast cancer using isosulfan blue dye. *J Womens Health* 1998;**7**:873–7.

29. Dale PS, Williams JT IV. Axillary staging utilizing selective sentinel lymphadenectomy for patients with invasive breast carcinoma. *Am Surg* 1998;**64**:28–31.

30. Kern KA. Sentinel lymph node mapping in breast cancer using subareolar injection of blue dye. *J Am Coll Surg* 1999;**189**:539–45.

31. Morgan A, Howisey RL, Aldape HC, et al. Initial experience in a community hospital with sentinel lymph node mapping and biopsy for evaluation of axillary lymph node status in palpable invasive breast cancer. *J Surg Oncol* 1999;**72**:24–31.

32. Morrow M, Rademaker AW, Bethke KP, et al. Leaning sentinel node biopsy: results of a prospective randomized trial of two techniques. *Surgery* 1999;**126**:714–22.

33. Albertini JJ, Lyman GH, Cox C, et al. Lymphatic mapping and sentinel node biopsy in the patient with breast cancer. *JAMA* 1996;**276**:1818–22.

34. Borgstein PJ, Meijer S, Pijpers R. Intradermal blue dye to identify sentinel lymph node in breast cancer. *Lancet* 1997;**349**:1668–9.

35. O'Hea BJ, Hill ADK, El-Shirbiny AM, et al. Sentinel lymph node biopsy in breast cancer: initial experience at Memorial Sloan-Kettering Cancer Center. *J Am Coll Surg* 1998;**186**:423–7.

36. Barnwell JM, Arredondo MA, Kollmorgen D, et al. Sentinel node biopsy in breast cancer. *Ann Surg Oncol* 1998;**5**:126–30.

37. Nwariaku FE, Euhus DM, Beitsch PD, et al. Sentinel lymph node biopsy, an alternative to elective axillary dissection for breast cancer. *Am J Surg* 1998;**176**:529–31.

38. Schneebaum S, Stadler J, Cohen M, et al. Gamma probe-guided sentinel node biopsy—optimal timing for injection. *Eur J Surg Oncol* 1998;**24**:515–19.

39. Canavese G, Gipponi M, Catturich A, et al. Sentinel lymph node mapping opens a new perspective in the surgical management of early-stage breast cancer: a combined approach with vital blue dye lymphatic mapping and radioguided surgery. *Semin Surg Oncol* 1998;**15**:272–7.

40. Czerniecki BJ, Scheff AM, Callans LS, et al. Immunohistochemistry with pancytokeratins improves the sensitivity of sentinel lymph node biopsy in patients with breast carcinoma. *Cancer* 1999;**85**:1098–1103.

41. van der Ent FWC, Kengen RAM, van der Pol HAG, et al. Sentinel node biopsy in 70 unselected patients with breast cancer: increased feasibility by using 10 mCi radiocolloid in combination with a blue dye tracer. *Eur J Surg Oncol* 1999;**25**:24–9.

42. Bass SS, Cox CE, Berman C, et al. The role of sentinel lymph node biopsy in breast cancer. *J Am Coll Surg* 1999;**189**:183–94.

43. Burak WE, Walker MJ, Yee LD, et al. Routine preoperative lymphoscintigraphy is not necessary prior to sentinel node biopsy for breast cancer. *Am J Surg* 1999;**177**:445–9.

44. Jaderborg JM, Harrison PB, Kiser JL, et al. The feasibility and accuracy of the sentinel lymph node biopsy for breast carcinoma. *Am Surg* 1999;**65**:699–705.

45. Turner RR. Histopathologic validation of the sentinel lymph node hypothesis for breast carcinoma. *Ann Surg* 1997;**226**:271–6.

46. Turner RR, Giuliano AE. Intraoperative pathologic examination of the sentinel lymph node. *Ann Surg* Oncol 1998;**5**:670–2.

47. Turner RR, Hansen NM, Stern SL, et al. Intraoperative examination of the sentinel lymph node for breast carcinoma staging. *Am J Clin Pathol* 1999;**112**:627–34.

48. Dowlatshahi K. Lymph node micrometastases from breast carcinoma: reviewing the dilemma. *Cancer* 1997;**80**:1188–97.

49. Prognostic importance of occult axillary lymph node micrometastases from breast cancers. International (Ludwig) Breast Cancer Study Group. *Lancet* 1990;**335**:1565–8.

50. Grube BJ, Giuliano AE. Observation of the breast cancer patient with a tumor-positive sentinel node: implications of the ACOSOG Z0011 trial. *Semin Surg Oncol* 2001;**20**:230–7.

51. Gemignani ML. Impact of sentinel lymph node mapping on relative charges in patients with early-stage breast cancer. *Ann Surg Oncol* 2000;**7**:575–80.

52. Hirsch JL. Use of isosulfan blue dye for identification of lymphatic vessels: experimental and clinical evidence. *Am J Roentgenol* 1982;**139**:1061–4.

53. Montgomery LL, Thorne AC, Van Zee KJ, et al. Isosulfan blue dye reactions during sentinel lymph node mapping for breast cancer. *Anesth Analg* 2002;**95**:385–8.

54. Kalimo K, Saarni H. Immediate reactions to patent blue dye. *Contact Dermatitis* 1981;**7**:171–2.

55. Mortazavi SH, Burrows BD. Allergic reaction to patient blue dye in lymphangiography. *Clin Radiol* 1971;**22**:389–90.

56. Linehan DC. Sentinel lymph node biopsy in breast cancer: unfiltered radioisotope is superior to filtered. *J Am Coll Surg* 1999;**188**:377–81.

57. Borgstein PJ, Meijer S, Pijpers RJ, et al. Functional lymphatic anatomy for sentinel node biopsy in breast cancer: echoes from the past and the periareolar blue method. *Ann Surg* 2000;**232**:81–9.

58. Hill AD, Tran KN, Akhurst T, et al. Lessons learned from 500 cases of lymphatic mapping for breast cancer. *Ann Surg* 1999;**229**:528–35.

59. McMasters KM, Tuttle TM, Carlson DJ, et al. Sentinel lymph node biopsy for breast cancer: a suitable alternative to routine axillary dissection in multi-institutional practice when optimal technique is used. *J Clin Oncol* 2000;**18**:2560–6.

60. Cody HS III. Sentinel lymph node mapping in breast cancer. *Oncology (Huntingt)* 1999;**13**:25–43.

61. Cody HS III, Borgen PI. State-of-the-art approaches to sentinel node biopsy for breast cancer: study design, patient selection, technique, and quality control at Memorial Sloan-Kettering Cancer Center. *Surg Oncol* 1999;**8**:85–91.

62. Gershenwald JE, Colome MI, Lee JE, et al. Patterns of recurrence following a negative sentinel lymph node biopsy in 243 patients with stage I or II melanoma. *J Clin Oncol* 1998;**16**:2253–60.

63. Chung MA, Steinhoff MM, Cady B. Clinical axillary recurrence in breast cancer patients after a negative sentinel node biopsy. *Am J Surg* 2002;**184**:310–14.

64. Blanchard DK, Donohue JH, Reynolds C, et al. Relapse and morbidity in patients undergoing sentinel lymph node biopsy alone or with axillary dissection for breast cancer. *Arch Surg* 2003;**138**:482–8.

65. Temple LK, Baron R, Cody HS 3rd, et al. Sensory morbidity after sentinel lymph node biopsy and axillary dissection: a prospective study of 233 women. *Ann Surg Oncol* 2002;**9**:654–62.

8 SENTINEL LYMPH NODE MAPPING IN ENDOMETRIAL CANCER

CHARLES LEVENBACK

BACKGROUND

Endometrial cancer is the most common gynecologic cancer in the USA with 39 300 cases reported in 2002.[1] Endometrial cancer is also one of the most curable gynecologic cancers. Although there is no screening test, the majority of patients present when the cancer is limited to the uterus. Early symptoms—in particular, postmenopausal bleeding—lead to early detection. For this reason, there were only 6300 deaths from endometrial cancer in the USA in 2002.[1]

Until the 1980s, most patients with endometrial cancer were treated with a combination of surgery and radiotherapy. Radiotherapy was commonly delivered prior to surgery, this sequence being preferred for a number of reasons. First, radiotherapy was thought to sterilize the lymph nodes and surgical bed: it was commonly believed that preoperative brachytherapy would prevent intraoperative dissemination caused by manipulation of the uterus during surgery. It was also believed that surgery might compromise the effectiveness of postoperative radiotherapy by interfering with tissue oxygenation in the surgical bed. Another reason preoperative radiotherapy was preferred is that it was feared that postoperative adhesions in the pelvis increased the risk of radiation enteritis and proctitis from postoperative radiotherapy. Once the pelvis was irradiated, there was no need for surgical treatment of the pelvic nodes.[2]

The standard of preoperative radiotherapy fell into disfavor in the early 1980s and has been abandoned for most patients. The primary reason is the recognition that preoperative radiotherapy resulted in the overtreatment of a large majority of patients. This was best demonstrated by Gynecologic Oncology Group trial 33, performed from 1977 to 1983. In this study, over 1000 patients with clinical stage I and II endometrial adenocarcinoma underwent complete surgical staging, including exploration of the abdominal cavity, peritoneal washings, selective pelvic and para-aortic lymph node sampling, and total abdominal hysterectomy and bilateral salpingo-oophorectomy. This study showed a clear relationship between lymph node metastases and depth of invasion. The rate of node metastases ranged from zero in patients with grade 1 tumors limited to the endometrium to 34% in patients with outer-third invasion and grade 3 tumors.[3] It was clear that patients at the lower end of the spectrum did not require node dissection, let alone radiotherapy.

The usefulness of postoperative radiotherapy in patients with intermediate or high-risk disease remains debatable. Three randomized trials have been conducted to examine this issue.[4-6] These studies show that radiotherapy reduces the risk of relapse within the field, but fail to show a consistent improvement in survival. These results have led some gynecologic oncologists to adopt a more aggressive surgical approach. This is exemplified by the work of Straughn et al,[7] who described a 5-year experience with complete pelvic and para-aortic lymphadenectomy along with total abdominal hysterectomy and bilateral salpingo-oophorectomy in patients with stage I endometrial cancer. Postoperative adjuvant radiotherapy was given to a small proportion of patients, primarily those with stage IC high-grade disease. The authors reported excellent survival rates for patients treated with this approach, including a 5-year overall survival rate of 96% for patients with intermediate-risk disease.

Others have pointed out that although this aggressive surgical approach does reduce the use of radiotherapy, aggressive surgery is associated with increased risk of bleeding, lymphedema, and, for patients who are irradiated, radiation enteritis.[8] Lymphatic mapping and sentinel node identification could be a way to identify node-positive patients without the morbidity of lymphadenectomy. The lymphatic mapping technique could be especially valuable in patients with comorbid conditions, in whom additional surgery clearly adds additional risks.

ENDOMETRIAL CANCER AS A TARGET FOR LYMPHATIC MAPPING

In the ideal lymphatic mapping situation, there is direct access to the tumor, allowing for peritumoral injection of blue dye or radionuclide. For example, in cutaneous melanoma, vulvar cancer, and cervix cancer, the lesion is both visible and palpable (Table 8.1), a fact which facilitates injection of dye or radionuclide. In breast cancer, the lesion is usually palpable but not visible, but in spite of this limitation, sentinel node identification has been very successful in breast cancer patients. Colon cancer is another model in which the primary tumor is not visible at laparotomy, but may be palpable, and there is interest

Table 8.1 Suitability of various tumors for lymphatic mapping.

Tumor	Tumor characteristics			
	Multiple lymphatic drainage basins	Clinically visible	Clinically palpable	Easy to inject with dye or radionuclide
Cutaneous melanoma	X	X	X	X
Breast cancer	X		X	X
Vulvar cancer		X	X	X
Cervix cancer		X	X	X
Colon cancer			X	X
Endometrial cancer	X			

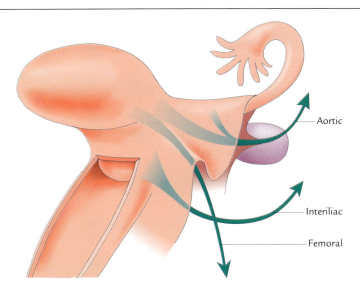

Figure 8.1   The most common lymphatic drainage pathways of the uterus are to iliac and para-aortic lymph nodes. Lymphatic drainage following the gonadal vessels can result in sentinel nodes at the level of the renal vessels. (Modified from Plentl and Friedman[9]).

in applying the sentinel node concept to this disease. Several authors have reported single-institution validation studies that appear to confirm the feasibility of lymphatic mapping in colorectal and other gastrointestinal tumors.[10–12] Feig et al,[13] however, have sounded a note of caution. They reported a false-negative rate of 38%, which is unacceptably high. In the case of endometrial cancer, the primary tumor cannot be seen, imaged, or palpated with standard clinical tools. Thus, endometrial cancer is a difficult target for the lymphatic mapping strategy.

One factor that makes the endometrium an attractive disease site for lymphatic mapping is the complexity of the lymphatic drainage of the uterus. Sentinel nodes can be found from the obturator space to the renal vessels (Figure 8.1).

LYMPHATIC MAPPING STUDIES IN ENDOMETRIAL CANCER PATIENTS

Several groups of investigators have studied lymphatic mapping and sentinel node identification in patients with endometrial cancer (Table 8.2). Echt et al[14] described their attempts at sentinel node identification in eight patients with endometrial cancer. Patent blue dye was injected into the uterine fundus at a depth of approximately half the thickness of the myometrium. The authors could not identify any sentinel nodes in any of the eight patients.

Burke et al[15] described intraoperative injection of isosulfan blue into the subserosal myometrium at three midline sites: at the fundus and at sites 2 cm anterior and 2 cm posterior to this site. These sites were chosen to mimic a fundal endometrial cancer. Dye uptake

Table 8.2 Published experiences with lymphatic mapping and sentinel node identification in patients with endometrial cancer.

First author, year	No. of cases	Location of injection	Radiotracer used?	Blue dye used?	Technical success rate*
Echt, 1999[14]	8	Myometrium	No	Yes	0%
Burke, 1996[15]	15	Subserosal	No	Yes	67%
Holub, 2002[17]	13	Subserosal	No	Yes	61%
	12	Subserosal and cervix	No	Yes	83%
Pelosi, 2002[18]	11	Cervix	Yes	Yes	Not stated
Niikura 2004[19]	28	Hysteroscopic	Yes	No	82%

* Technical success was defined as identification of at least one sentinel node.

was seen in the lymphatic channels and lymph nodes within 10 min. Blue-stained nodes were identified, and their location recorded. The nodes were sent for pathology review as separate specimens. A selective pelvic and para-aortic lymphadenectomy was then performed. Blue dye was deposited in lymph nodes in 10 of 15 patients. Blue nodes were found in the pelvic and para-aortic areas (Figure 8.2). Blue nodes were not found between the bifurcation of the aorta and the origin of the inferior mesenteric artery. This confirms the observation of many anatomists that the lymphatic drainage of the uterus follows two paths, along the uterine vessels to the pelvis and along the gonadal vessels to the para-aortics at the level of the renal vessels. Four patients had positive lymph nodes. The blue-stained nodes were positive in two patients. One patient with bulky nodes had no dye uptake, and one patient had a micrometastasis to an unstained node in the obturator space.

Holub and colleagues[16] described a laparoscopic-assisted technique for lymphatic mapping in patients with endometrial cancer. The eight patients in their series underwent intraoperative injection of blue dye at the same locations described by Burke et al, injections being given with a 5-mm laparoscopic puncture needle. Blue nodes were found in the obturator, internal iliac, and common iliac sites in 11 lymph nodes among five patients.

Holub et al later expanded on their experience and reported on two techniques for lymphatic mapping in endometrial cancer in 2002.[17] In this study, 13 patients underwent subserosal injection, as described in the first report, and 12 patients underwent both subserosal and cervical injections. With the addition of cervical injections, the rate of observation of blue-stained lymph nodes increased from 61.5% in the group to 83.3%. The authors suggested that the combined approach was superior.

Pelosi et al[18] described using a combination of radioactive tracer and blue dye in 11 patients with early endometrial cancer during laparoscopic-assisted vaginal hysterectomy and bilateral salpingo-oophorectomy. The tracer and blue dye were injected into the cervix. Three sentinel nodes were identified that proved to be positive for micrometastases.

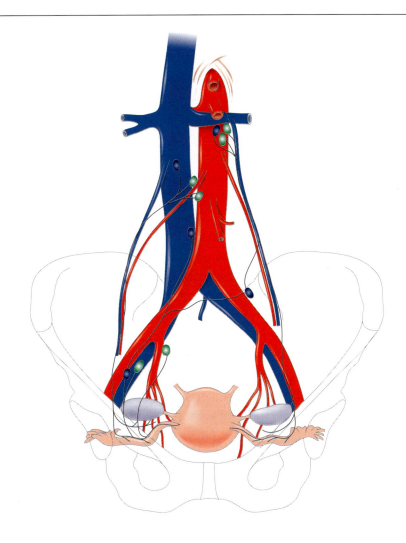

Figure 8.2 Location of sentinel lymph nodes of the uterus. Note that para-aortic sentinel nodes were found above the inferior mesenteric artery.[15]

At the University of Texas M.D. Anderson Cancer Center, we have been conducting a clinical trial of intraoperative lymphoscintigraphy in patients with endometrial cancer. In this ongoing trial, we are injecting radionuclide into the fundus at the locations used for the aforementioned blue dye studies. Intraoperative lymphoscintigrams are obtained with a portable gamma camera. The results of these efforts will be reported soon.

The most important recent development is a report of sentinel node identification utilizing hysteroscopically guided injection of radiolabeled technetium-99m phytate the day before hysterectomy.[19] When possible, injections were made in four locations around the tumor. In patients who had complete involvement of the endometrial cavity, five standard sites were injected. Lymphoscintigrams were obtained following the injection and then again the next morning, prior to surgery. Intraoperative localization was performed with a hand-held gamma probe. At least one sentinel node was identified in 23 (82%) of 28 patients. The results were best (21 out of 22) among the patients with invasion limited to the inner 50% of the myometrium. Six patients had invasion greater than 50%; sentinel nodes were identified in only four of these patients. Fifteen patients had sentinel nodes in both pelvic and para-aortic locations; five patients had sentinel nodes in pelvic locations only; and, a finding not described before, three patients had sentinel nodes in para-aortic sites only. Only one patient of the 16 in whom sentinel nodes were identified had metastases.

This hysteroscopically guided technique is an improvement over techniques that rely on injection into the uterine fundus or cervix without visualization of the actual tumor. In addition, this technique provides a preoperative lymphoscintigram that can be helpful for planning the operative procedure. The most cephalad sentinel node can be identified and perhaps a determination can be made about how long an incision will be required to reach it. A drawback of this new technique is that it requires another procedure and a 2-day sequence. It remains to be seen whether other groups can replicate these results. In addition, questions remain about the safety of hysteroscopy in patients with endometrial cancer. Is it safe to irrigate the uterus and possibly spill cancer cells into the pelvis? How much, if any, radioactive material finds its way into the pelvis and onto drapes and sponges during the laparotomy?

SUMMARY

Endometrial cancer has proved to be a difficult disease site in which to perform lymphatic mapping and sentinel node identification. The uterus has complex lymphatic drainage, with sentinel nodes potentially far from the primary tumor at the level of renal vessels or in the groin. This makes endometrial cancer an appealing target for lymphatic mapping; however, multiple technical challenges remain before mapping can be reliably performed in endometrial cancer patients.

REFERENCES

1. Jemal A, Thomas A, Murray T, et al. Cancer statistics, 2002. *CA Cancer J Clin* 2002;**52**:23–47.
2. Starreveld AA, Shankowsky HA, Koch M. Canadian Association of Radiologists: treatment results in 2719 patients with carcinoma of the endometrium 1973–1977. *Can Assoc Radiol J* 1987;**38**:96–105.
3. Creasman W, Morrow CP, Bundy BN, et al. Surgical pathologic spread patterns of endometrial cancer: a Gynecologic Oncology Group study. *Cancer* 1987;**60**:2035–41.

4. Aalders J, Abeler V, Kolstad P, et al. Postoperative external irradiation and prognostic parameters in stage I endometrial carcinoma. *Obstet Gynecol* 1980;**56**:419–27.

5. Roberts WS, Kavanagh JJ, Greenberg H, et al. Concomitant radiation therapy and chemotherapy in the treatment of advanced squamous carcinoma of the lower female genital tract. *Gynecol Oncol* 1989;**34**:183–6.

6. Creutzberg CL, Van Putten WL, Koper PC, et al. Surgery and postoperative radiotherapy versus surgery alone for patients with stage-1 endometrial carcinoma: multicentre randomised trial. PORTEC Study Group. Post Operative Radiation Therapy in Endometrial Carcinoma. *Lancet* 2000;**355**(9213):1404–11.

7. Straughn JM, Huh WK, Kelly FJ, et al. Conservative management of stage I endometrial carcinoma after surgical staging. *Gynecol Oncol* 2002;**84**:194–200.

8. Russell AH. No regrets, no illusions. *Gynecol Oncol* 2002;**84**:191–3.

9. Plentl AA, Friedman EA. Lymphatics of the cervix uteri. In: *Lymphatic System of Female Genitalia* (WB Saunders: Philadelphia, 1971) 75–115.

10. Saha S, Nora D, Wong JH, et al. Sentinel lymph node mapping in colorectal cancer—a review. *Surg Clin North Am* 2000;**80**:1811–19.

11. Lin KM, Rodriguez F, Ota DM. The sentinel node in colorectal carcinoma. Mapping technique, pathologic assessment, and clinical relevance. *Oncology (Huntingt)* 2002;**16**:567–75, 580; discussion, 580, 582, 585.

12. Tsioulias GJ, Wood TF, Morton DL, et al. Lymphatic mapping and focused analysis of sentinel lymph nodes upstage gastrointestinal neoplasms. *Arch Surg* 2000;**135**:926–32.

13. Feig BW, Curley S, Lucci A, et al. A caution regarding lymphatic mapping in patients with colon cancer. *Am J Surg* 2001;**182**:707–12.

14. Echt M, Finan MA, Hoffman MS, et al. Detection of sentinel lymph nodes with lymphazurin in cervical, uterine, and vulvar malignancies. *South Med J* 1999;**92**:204–8.

15. Burke TW, Levenback C, Tornos C, et al. Intraabdominal lymphatic mapping to direct selective pelvic and paraaortic lymphadenectomy in women with high-risk endometrial cancers: results of a pilot study. *Gynecol Oncol* 1996;**62**:169–73.

16. Holub Z, Kliment L, Lukac J, et al. Laparoscopically-assisted intraoperative lymphatic mapping in endometrial cancer: preliminary results. *Eur J Gynaecol Oncol* 2001;**22**:118–21.

17. Holub Z, Jabor A, Kliment L. Comparison of two procedures for sentinel lymph node detection in patients with endometrial cancer: a pilot study. *Eur J Gynaecol Oncol* 2002;**23**:53–7.

18. Pelosi E, Arena V, Baudino B, et al. Preliminary study of sentinel node identification with 99mTc colloid and blue dye in patients with endometrial cancer. *Tumori* 2002;**88**:S9–S10.

19. Niikura H, Okamura C, Utsunomiya H, et al. Sentinel lymph node detection in patients with endometrial cancer. *Gynecol Oncol* 2004;**92**:669–74.

9 DIFFUSION OF INNOVATION AND CLINICAL TRIAL DESIGN IN LYMPHATIC MAPPING

CHARLES LEVENBACK

DIFFUSION OF INNOVATION

Lymphatic mapping and sentinel node identification are commonly described as the most important innovations in surgical management of solid tumors since Halsted described radical mastectomy with en bloc lymphadenectomy.[1] Gould et al[2] are credited with the first use of the term 'sentinel lymph node' in the 1960s, yet it took over 30 years for the procedure to be refined and popularized. Even now, definitive data to support sentinel node biopsy alone as an alternative to lymphadenectomy are lacking.

What has taken so long? In fact, as shown by Everett Rogers in *Diffusion of Innovations*, diffusion of innovation, medical and otherwise, often occurs slowly. In 1601, Captain John Lancaster of the Royal Navy left England with four ships bound for India. On one of the ships, the sailors were given normal rations; on the other ships, they were given normal rations plus 3 tablespoons of lemon juice a day. The mortality rate from scurvy was dramatically lower in the 'experimental' group than the 'control' group. Definitive results like this are rare in clinical trials, yet the Admiralty largely ignored the results. Other factors, such as budgets, politics, innovations in arms and navigation, and war fighting, were higher priorities for the leadership. Opinion leaders such as Captain James Cook, who explored the Pacific, were skeptical of Lancaster's results. It took almost 200 years and several other studies with similar results to make citrus supplements mandatory for all sailors in the Royal Navy. Scurvy was eradicated almost immediately after citrus supplements were instituted.[3]

More recently, the value of other innovations has at times been overlooked. In the 1970s, a research team at Xerox Corporation developed the personal computer, with a mouse, icons, pull-down menus, and a laser printer, yet it was another company, Apple Computer, that brought these innovations to the marketplace, and yet another company, Microsoft, that successfully dominated the software segment of the market. The leadership at Xerox saw the company as a copier company, not a computer company.[3] Sometimes new innovations are blocked by investment in the status quo. The so-called QWERTY keyboard now in universal use was designed to *slow down* typists, who would jam the early mechanical models if they typed too fast. More rational keyboards for the electronic age have been designed; however, they are resisted by manufacturers, trainers, and typists who are already familiar with the QWERTY design.

In medicine, there have been recent attempts to accelerate acceptance of innovation. Consensus panels and conferences are common. The National Cancer Institute issued a clinical announcement in 1999[4] to discuss the results of several clinical trials that showed a survival advantage for patients treated with chemoradiation compared with radiation alone for advanced cervix cancer. Three of the trials were published simultaneously in the *New England Journal of Medicine*. Simultaneous publications and a clinical alert backed by the prestige of the National Cancer Institute probably accelerated the adoption of chemoradiation as a standard treatment compared to the speed with which it would have been adopted after traditional forms of communication.

Diffusion of lymphatic mapping was slow between 1960 and 1992. In 1992, Morton et al[5] described the use of lymphoscintigraphy and blue dye in melanoma patients. At this time, there was controversy within the melanoma community regarding the merits of regional lymphadenectomy. Lymphatic mapping appeared to offer a solution to many of the problems with regional lymphadenectomy, and melanoma physicians rapidly embraced the new procedure. It was a short leap from melanoma to breast cancer. In the 1990s, there was rapid growth in the number of clinical trials and publications regarding lymphatic mapping.

THE IMPORTANCE AND PROPER DESIGN OF CLINICAL TRIALS

Clinical trials in medicine are frequent drivers of innovation. Published data are commented on and debated at all levels of organized medicine. Frequently, there are many interpretations of the same set of facts. Continued learning is a valued and frequently mandatory aspect of the life of clinicians, and review of clinical trial results is a primary component of this continued learning.

INSTITUTIONAL REVIEW BOARD APPROVAL AND INFORMED CONSENT

It is important to observe well-established guidelines for trial design. Modern clinical trials require approval by an institutional review board. This body, which includes physicians, scientists, statisticians, and laypersons, is subject to review by governmental agencies. Trials that have governmental funding are likely to be reviewed at a national or at least a regional level. Investigators commonly find this process overbearing; however, it is wise to remember that the system is, in part, a result of unethical treatment of patients by the medical establishment in the past. The current systems protect not only the patients but also the physicians. Clinical investigators are wise to stay within the bounds of established national and local policy and procedure.

Nevertheless, breakthroughs can and do occur outside the strict interpretation of these policies and procedures. The first modern description of lymphatic mapping, penile lymphography, by Riveros et al,[6] was performed in a group of indigent patients, some with penile carcinoma and some without. Published reports of subsequent trials have not always specified that institutional review board approval and informed consent were obtained. As a general principle, if a clinician intends to gather data and publish them, a protocol should be written and consent obtained. New guidelines are in place that require institutional review board approval for retrospective studies of clinical management and outcomes, even if the requirement of individual informed consent from patients is waived.

STATISTICS

Valid statistical definitions and design are crucial to the success of clinical trials. Protocols require a statistical section, and institutional reviews almost always include a statistician. Feasibility trials usually include small numbers of patients and look at only a few descriptive statistics, such as the technical success rate. Validation trials usually include more patients and report statistics such as sensitivity, specificity, and negative predictive value. Statistics commonly reported in clinical trials of lymphatic mapping are listed in Table 9.1.

Table 9.1 Statistics commonly reported in clinical trials of lymphatic mapping.

Measure	How calculated *	Notes
False-negative rate	false-negative ÷ true-positive	Rate is calculated on the basis of node-positive patients only
Sensitivity	true-positive ÷ true-positive + false-negative	Proportion of node-positive patients with positive SLN
Negative predictive value	True-negative ÷ True-negative + false-negative	Proportion of node-negative patients with negative SNL
Technical success rate	no. of patients in whom SLN identified Total number of patients	May be calculated for lymph node basins—i.e., no. of basins in which SLN identified/total no. of basins examined
Accuracy	true-positive + true-negative ÷ total	Proportion of cases in which SLN identified in which SLN status correlated with status of lymph node basin

* 'True-positive', 'true-negative', and 'false-negative' indicated total number of patients with such a finding on SLN biopsy and regional lymphadenectomy.
SLN: sentinel lymph node.

Studies frequently report the rate of false-negative sentinel nodes. This is calculated on the basis of node-positive patients only, not on the basis of all patients in whom sentinel nodes are identified.

Randomized trials require more detailed statistical design. These trials require a rational hypothesis and the statistical power to answer the questions posed by the hypothesis. These trials are likely to look beyond technical success, sensitivity, and negative predictive value to more common oncologic outcome measures, such as progression-free survival and overall survival. Various statistical measures are required to compare two or more treatment plans. In the past, randomized trials have focused on survival outcomes alone. Modern studies should include data regarding the complication rates of various treatments as well as quality of life.

PRECLINICAL TRIALS

There have been very few preclinical trials regarding lymphatic mapping. The most important was by Wong,[7] who described the characteristics of various dyes in a feline model. Mapping procedures have been associated with very low surgical risk to individual patients, making extensive animal modeling unnecessary.

FEASIBILITY TRIALS

As the name implies, the purpose of a feasibility trial is to determine whether a procedure can be performed in human subjects. It is unwise for investigators to perform new unestablished procedures, even diagnostic procedures, without the protection of a clinical trial. These protocols usually require only a brief description and rationale for the procedure and minimal, if any, statistical input. Data from feasibility trials[5,8–10] provided the rationale background section for future, larger validation trials.

VALIDATION TRIALS

Validation trials aim to provide basic descriptive statistics regarding sensitivity, specificity, positive and negative predictive value, complication rates, and other insights into the new procedure. In validation trials of lymphatic mapping, sentinel node identification is followed by regional lymphadenectomy. Numerous validation trials were initiated in melanoma and breast cancer following the initial feasibility trials. In the case of breast cancer, these trials ranged in size from a few dozen patients to hundreds. These studies tended to be single-institution trials, and there were numerous variations on the general mapping theme. For example, the general definition of the sentinel node as the first draining lymph

Table 9.2 (Reprint from Cody,[18] p 98 with permission from Martin Dunitz).

Proposed 'standard' definitions of radioactive SLNs. Radioactive SLNs have been defined by various methods and by a variety of investigators. The range of definitions may relate to the differences in techniques employed by each surgeon.	
Investigator	**Definition of SLN**
Krag et al (1995)	15 counts/10 s plus in vivo node/background ratio ≥ 3
Pijpers et al (1995)	Node with highest counts
Mudun et al (1996)	300–3000 counts/10 s plus in vivo node/bckground ratio ≥ 3
Albertini et al (1996)	In vivo node/background ratio ≥ 2
Thompson et al (1997)	Node/residual basin background ratio ≥ 3
Bostick et al (1997)	In vivo node/background ratio ≥ 2
Leong et al (1997)	In vivo node/backgound ratio ≥ 3
Essner et al (2000)	In vivo node/background ratio ≥ 2
Murray et al (2000)	Node with highest counts
Jansen et al (2000)	Node with highest counts

node is the same in all of these trials; however, the precise criteria for a positive sentinel node varied from study to study (Table 9.2). Some studies used blue dye or radiocolloid for sentinel node identification, whereas others used both. Typically, these studies involved a relatively small number of surgeons, allowing analysis of the so-called learning curve and variations between individual surgeons.[11,12] In gynecologic oncology, progress with validation trials of lymphatic mapping has been slow since the number of available patients at any one institution is small and therefore accrual is slow. Sometimes several institutions can work together to accelerate accrual.[13]

In the case of vulvar cancer, the disease is so rare that the only practical way to gather enough data is through the multi-institutional cooperative groups. This process requires consensus building and multiple levels of approval that can take years to achieve. On the other hand, multi-institutional research groups provide funding for their members, the opportunity to learn the procedure with the protection of the protocol, and, hopefully, a wide audience for the results. The ultimate goal of new procedures is wide application, not single-institution use. Multi-institutional groups determine whether a procedure can be performed successfully in multiple setting with different physicians, consultants, and resources.

OBSERVATIONAL TRIALS

Observational trials are relatively uncommon; however, they can play a big role in the development of a new procedure. These studies have an 'experimental' arm without comparison to a 'standard' treatment arm. A rare tumor, such as vulvar cancer, is an especially appealing site for observational studies, since such studies require far fewer patients than a randomized trial and multiple validation trials have already been published.

An observational trial of the efficacy of staging by the sentinel lymph node procedure in vulvar cancer is under way in the Netherlands. There are 200 new cases of vulvar cancer a year in the Netherlands, so it is easy to see that a randomized trial would be impractical in this environment. The investigators have published their validation data[14] and decided to proceed with this observation trial. Every effort is being made in this study to avoid false-negative sentinel nodes, which might result in relapse. Case selection is careful and limited to patients with T1 and T2 lesions less than 4 cm in size. Sentinel nodes are identified by using both radiocolloid and blue dye. Extensive ultrastaging of the sentinel node is carried out with serial sectioning and immunohistochemical staining. Patients with sentinel node metastases found at any time are taken off the study, and subjected to full inguinal femoral lymphadenectomy. The statistical design includes interim data analysis and early stopping rules based on the number of groin recurrences observed.

RANDOMIZED TRIALS

Randomized trials can have a profound impact on medical practice. They usually involve a direct comparison between a standard treatment and a new or experimental treatment. Randomized trials have occasionally proved observational trials to be incorrect.[15] If the experimental treatment proves to be superior, it replaces the old standard treatment and becomes the new standard. Randomized trials frequently require a large patient population, external funding, and the support of a multi-institutional group. Since these trials involve so many resources and investigators, the design of the trial usually represents a consensus of opinion and compromise on various factors. Since these studies are the result of a political process, the scientific integrity of the trials is sometimes questioned by purists. In spite of theses compromises and shortcomings, randomized trials are the most likely to generate acceptance of innovation.

The first randomized trials to incorporate lymphatic mapping were for patients with early melanoma. The Multicenter Selective Lymphadenectomy Trial was initiated in 1995 in 16 centers. The study is open to patients with invasive melanoma 1 mm in thickness or more who are good surgical candidates. The goal of the study is to determine whether sentinel lymph node biopsy with completion lymphadenectomy for sentinel-node-positive patients will improve survival compared with wide local excision alone (Figure 9.1). This study has a skill-verification feature that requires at least 85% accuracy among 30 patients who undergo mapping. The study provides for the mapping technique (blue dye and

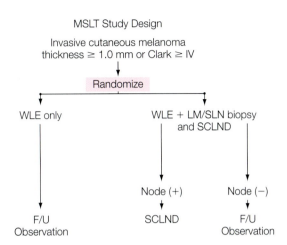

Figure 9.1 The Multicenter Selective Lymphadenectomy Trial (primary end-point overall survival). WLE: wide-local excision; LM/SLN biopsy: lymphatic mapping and sentinel lymph-node biopsy SCLND: selective complete lymph-node dissection; F/U: follow-up. (After Morton et al,[16] with permission from Martin Dunitz.)

radiocolloid) as well as pathologic ultrastaging of the sentinel node. As of the last report in 1999,[16] over 1000 patients had been entered, and the technical success rate was over 95%.

The Sunbelt Melanoma Trial, opened in 1997, has eligibility requirements similar to those of the multicenter selective lymphadenectomy trial: patients must have melanoma 1 mm or thicker and be candidates for wide local excision (Figure 9.2). All patients undergo sentinel lymph node biopsy. Histologic analysis of the sentinel nodes includes serial sectioning with hematoxylin-eosin (HE) staining and polymerase chain reaction (PCR) testing for melanoma DNA if the standard histologic testing is negative for tumor. Patients with a positive sentinel lymph node on histologic testing undergo regional lymphadenectomy. If the sentinel node is the only positive lymph node, patients are randomized to observation or 1 year of alpha-interferon treatments. If findings on histologic testing and PCR analysis are negative, the patients are observed. If histologic findings are negative and PCR findings are positive, patients are randomized to observation, regional lymphadenectomy, or 1 year of alpha-interferon. Around 3000 patients will have to be enrolled to complete the study (Figure 9.2). The Sunbelt Melanoma Trial draws a distinction between tumors with ambiguous lymphatic drainage patterns and those with predictable patterns. Preoperative lymphoscintigraphy is required if the primary tumor is at a site with ambiguous drainage. Intraoperative lymphoscintigraphy is performed on all patients. The use of blue dye is recommended but not mandatory.

The National Surgical Adjuvant Breast and Bowel Project (NSABP) B-32 trial (Figure 9.3) is based on the hypothesis that sentinel node biopsy alone will produce the same outcomes in terms of staging and survival as axillary lymphadenectomy, but with reduced morbidity. The protocol requires the use of both blue dye and radiocolloid, and sentinel nodes are subjected to serial sectioning and routine HE staining. Immunohistochemical analysis is

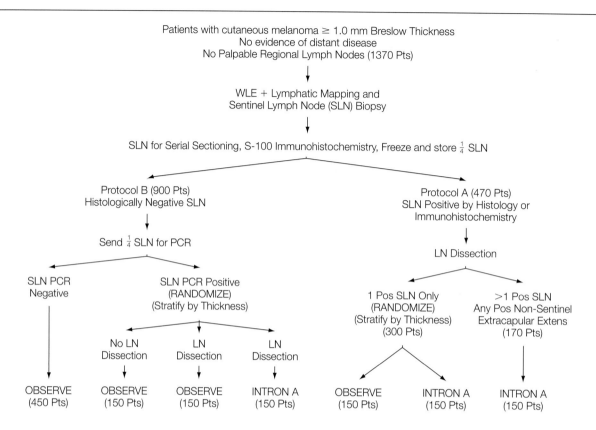

Figure 9.2 The Sunbelt Melanoma Trial.

used only to confirm suspected micrometastases seen on HE staining. There are no treatment elements to the study; however, complications are carefully documented, and quality of life surveys are performed (Figure 9.3). This study approaches the question, 'Is there an acceptable increase in mortality for a reduction in morbidity?' An interactive poll taken at a meeting of the American Society of Breast Surgeons found that respondents overwhelmingly believed that it is not acceptable to allow mortality to rise to reduce the morbidity of axillary lymphadenectomy.[15] The NSABP study will help determine the price in mortality, if any, of reduced surgical morbidity.

The most ambitious trials are the American College of Surgeons Z-0010 (Figure 9.4) and Z-0011 (Figure 9.5) protocols. The Z-0010 study is for patients with clinical stage I or II breast cancer amenable to breast-conserving surgery. The objectives are to determine the incidence and significance of micrometastases to the sentinel node and bone marrow on the basis of immunohistochemical staining and to evaluate the risk of regional relapse following sentinel node biopsy only when the node is negative on routine histologic evaluation. Following registration, all patients undergo breast-conserving surgery, sentinel node biopsy, and iliac crest bone marrow aspiration. Sentinel-node-negative patients have no specific axillary treatment, though they can receive breast radiotherapy or systemic adjuvant therapy as appropriate on the basis of other prognostic factors (Figure 9.4). Sentinel-node-positive patients are eligible for the Z-0011 study and are randomized to no further

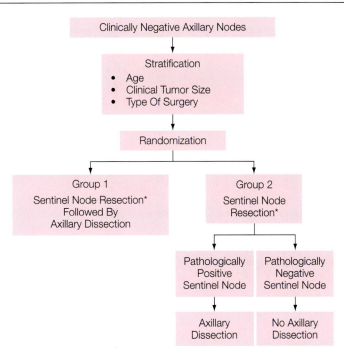

Figure 9.3 The National Surgical Adjuvant Breast and Bowel Project B-32 trial protocol schema.

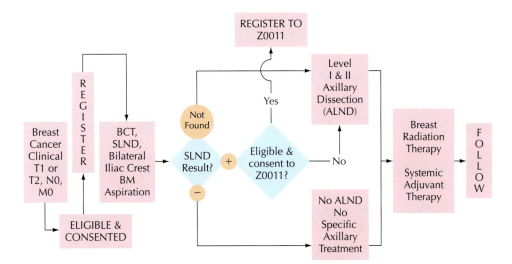

Figure 9.4 American College of Surgeons Z-0010 protocol schema
Reprinted with permission from the American College of Surgeons Oncology Group, Protocol Z-0010. The conduct of this protocol was supported by Grant Number 5U10 CA76001-5 from the National Caller Institute (NCI). The contents of this text are solely the responsibility of the authors and do not necessarily represent the official views of the NCI.

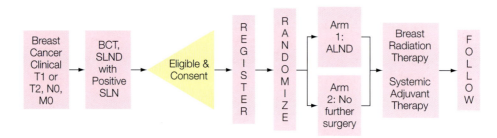

Figure 9.5   Americal College of Surgeons Z-0011 protocol schema
Reprinted with permission from the American College of Surgeons Oncology Group, Protocol Z-0011. The conduct of this protocol was supported by Grant Number 5U10 CA76001-5 from the National Caller Institute (NCI). The contents of this text are solely the responsibility of the authors and do not necessarily represent the official views of the NCI.

axillary treatment or axillary lymphadenectomy. All patients may receive breast radiotherapy or systemic adjuvant therapy as appropriate (Figure 9.5). The study has been amended since it was opened to make the bone marrow aspiration mandatory and to open Z-0011 to patients not on Z-0010. The final accrual will probably reach over 8000 patients, with close to 3500 bone marrow samples being sent to a central reference laboratory.

The Z-0010 study has a surgeon-skill-verification requirement. A case list of 20 cases per surgeon must be submitted before the surgeon can participate. Individuals can substitute verification from a participating institution that they received training in the technique during a residency or fellowship. The protocol allows for the use of blue dye, radiocolloid, or both to identify sentinel nodes.

RANDOMIZED TRIALS IN GYNECOLOGIC CANCER

At present, there are no randomized trials of lymphatic mapping in gynecologic cancer; however, there are attempts to develop such a study in vulvar cancer both in North America and Europe. The vulvar cancer model poses several challenges. The regional relapse rate following sentinel node biopsy only must be very low for the procedure to gain acceptance among gynecologic oncologists. In addition, debate persists over the therapeutic value of regional lymphadenectomy versus, for example, regional radiotherapy.[17] Concepts under consideration include randomization of sentinel-node-negative patients to observation or completion lymphadenectomy. Sentinel-node-positive patients could be randomized to completion lymphadenectomy or regional radiotherapy (or chemoradiation). The results of the Netherlands observational trial and GOG 173 will assist in designing a randomized trial that will enjoy widespread support.

REFERENCES

1. Halsted W. The results of radical operations for the cure of carcinoma of the breast. *Ann Surg* 1907;**46**:1.

2. Gould E, Winship T, Philbin PH, et al. Observations on a 'sentinel node' in cancer of the parotid. *Cancer* 1960;**13**:77–8.

3. Rogers E. *Diffusion of Innovations* 4th edn (Free Press: New York, 1995) 518.

4. NCI. *Concurrent Chemoradiation for Cervical Cancer* (National Institutes of Health, Washington, DC, 1999).

5. Morton DL, Wen DR, Wong JH, et al. Technical details of intraoperative lymphatic mapping for early stage melanoma. *Arch Surg* 1992;**127**:392–9.

6. Riveros M, Garcia R, Cabanas R. Lymphadenography of the dorsal lymphatics of the penis. Technique and results. *Cancer* 1967;**20**:2026–31.

7. Wong JH. Lymphatic drainage of skin in a sentinel lymph node in a feline model. *Ann Surg* 1991;**214**:637–41.

8. Krag DN, Meijer SJ, Weaver DL, et al. Minimal-access surgery for staging of malignant melanoma. *Arch surg* 1995;**130**:654–8; discussion 659–660.

9. Levenback C, Burke TW, Gershenson DM, et al. Intraoperative lymphatic mapping for vulvar cancer. *Obstet Gynecol* 1994;**84**:163–7.

10. O'Boyle J, Coleman RL, Bernstein SG, et al. Intraoperative lymphatic mapping in cervix cancer patients undergoing radical hysterectomy: a pilot study. *Gynecol Oncol* 2000;**79**:238–43.

11. Cody HS, Hill ADK, Tran KN, et al. Credentialing for breast lymphatic mapping: how many cases are enough? *Ann Surg* 1999;**229**:723–8.

12. Krag D, Weaver D, Ashikaga T, et al. The sentinel node in breast cancer. *N Engl J Med* 1998;**339**:941–6.

13. Levenback C, Coleman RL, Burke TW, et al. Intraoperative lymphatic mapping of the vulva with blue dye. In: *31st Annual Meeting of the Society of Gynecologic Oncologists* (*Gynecologic Oncology*: San Diego, CA, 2000).

14. de Hullu JA, Hollema H, Piers DA, et al. Sentinel lymph node procedure is highly accurate in squamous cell carcinoma of the vulva. *J Clin Oncol* 2000;**18**:2811–16.

15. Krag D. Why perform randomized clinical trials for sentinel node surgery for breast cancer? *Am J Surg* 2001;**182**:411–13.

16. Morton DL, Thompson JF, Essner R, et al. Validation of the accuracy of intraoperative lymphatic mapping and sentinel lymphadenectomy for early-stage melanoma: a multicenter trial. Multicenter Selective Lymphadenectomy Trial Group. *Ann Surg* 1999;**230**:453–63; discussion 463–5.

17. Katz A, Eifel P, Jhingran A, et al. Role of radiation therapy in reducing regional recurrences of invasive squamous cell carcinoma of the vulva. *Int J Radiat Oncol Biol Phys* 2003;**57**:409–18.

18. Cody HS. *Sentinel Lymph Node Biopsy* (Martin Dunitz: London, 2002) 370.

INDEX

Page numbers in italics indicate tables and figures. SLN refers to sentinal lymph nodes.

abdominal lymphatics, early drawings *2*
absorbance spectra of vital dyes *72*
AE1/3 91
allergic reactions to blue dyes 70–1, 142, 160
American College of Surgeons Oncology Group
    (ACOSOG) trials, breast cancer 158–9,
    186–8, *187*, *188*
American Joint Committee on Cancer (AJCC)
    staging for breast cancer 149–52, *149–51*, *152*
anastomosis of Poirier 51
antibodies, breast cancer immunohistochemistry
    90–1
antimony sulfide 20
aortic lymph node metastases
    endometrial cancer 52–3
    ovarian cancer 56
axilla
    blood supply 59
    lymph nodes *62*, *153*
      classification 60, *63*
      dissection 60, *63*, 152–3
      SLN identification 63–4, *64*
    nerves 60
axillary artery 59

blue dyes
    dyes assessed 68, *68*, *69*
    early in vivo injection studies 5–7
    mapping techniques 69–70
      applicability 80
      efficacy 78–9
      see also specific cancers
    safety 70–2, *72*, 142, 160
brachytherapy, cervix cancer 125, 128
Braithwaite, L. 17
breast
    anatomy 59
    blood supply 60, *61*
    lymphatics 60
    lymph nodes 60, *62*, *63*
breast cancer
    Halsted surgical approach *4*
    lifetime risk 147
    micrometastases, clinical significance 158

models of spread 17–18, *18*
natural history 147
pathology 147–9, *148*
staging 149–52, *149–51*, *152*
breast cancer, SLN mapping 153–67
    contraindications 154, 158
    follow-up 166
    indications 154
    intraoperative techniques 159–60
    learning curve 161
    morbidity 166
    pathologic analysis
      fine-needle aspiration cytology 91
      frozen section analysis 86
      immunohistochemistry 90–1, 158, *159*
      imprint cytology 87
      RT-PCR 92
    procedure
      preoperative lymphoscintigraphy 162, *162*
      blue dye injection 162, *163*, *164*
      identification/removal of nodes 162, *165*, *166*
    suitability *172*
    technical issues
      blue dyes 160
      radioisotopes 161
    validation studies 154, *155–7*

Cabanas, Ramon 7–9, *8*
cadaver studies of lymphatic anatomy 1–3, *2*, *3*
CAM5.2 90
cancer
    early models 3
    suitability for lymphatic mapping *172*
    see also specific cancers
cardinal ligaments 42, *42*
cats, lymphatic drainage 68
CEA 91
cervical lymphatics
    early studies 2, *3*, *6*
    topographic anatomy 43, *130*
      anterior trunks 46
      lateral trunks 43–4, *44*, 134, *135*
      posterior trunks 45, *45*, 134, *136*
cervix, topographic anatomy 41–2, *41*, *42*

cervix cancer
  human papillomavirus infections 125–6, 142–3
  incidence and mortality 125
  lymph node metastases
    likelihood 46, 47
    orderly occurrence 130
    and prognosis 128, 129
  management
    advanced disease 127
    cancer evaluation 126–7
    chemoradiation 128, 130
    historical 125
    local medical resources 129
    surgery 128
  molecular biology of SLNs 142–3
  natural history 46–7
  risk factors 126
  stages 127
cervix cancer, SLN mapping 69–70
  allergy to blue dyes 142
  clinical experience
    blue dye alone 135–6, 138–9
    laparoscopy with combined technique 140–2,
      141
    lymphoscintigraphy 79, 139–40, 140
    published trials summarized 137
  future development 143
  operator experience 142
  RT-PCR studies of cytokeratin 19 93, 143
  suitability 129–31, 129, 172
  technique
    blue dye mapping 132–5, 133, 134, 135, 136
    lymphoscintigraphy 77, 131–2, 132
clinical trial design 180–8
  institutional review board approval 180–1
  statistics 181–2, 182
  trial types
    feasibility 182
    observational 184
    preclinical 182
    randomized see randomized clinical trials
    validation 182–3, 183
Cloquet's node 30, 32
colloids see radiocolloids
colon cancer, suitability for lymphatic mapping
  172–3, 172
corpus uteri 49–54
  endometrial cancer see endometrial cancer

lymphatic anatomy
  capillaries 50
  channels 51–2, 51
  regional nodes 52
  SLNs 175
  subserosal network 50–1, 50
cutaneous melanoma see melanoma: cutaneous
cyalume 68
cytokeratin 19 93, 143
cytotoxic T cells, microenvironment and
  activation 23

deep inguinal lymphatics 32, 33
dendritic cells, in SLNs 23
diffusion of innovation 179–80
DiSaia, Philip 9, 37
DNA flow cytometry (DNA FCM) 91–2
ductal carcinoma in situ, breast (DCIS) 147, 148
dyes see blue dyes

Eichner, Eduard 7
EMA 90–1
endocervix 42
endometrial cancer
  lymph node metastases 49, 52–3, 171
  radiotherapy 171–2
  surgery 171, 172
endometrial cancer, SLN mapping 171–7
  blue dye 53, 70, 173–4
  hysteroscopically guided technique 175–6
  intraoperative lymphoscintigraphy 175
  radiotracer and blue dye 53, 174
  studies summarized 174
  suitability 172–3, 172, 173
endometrial lymphatics 50
exocervix 41–2

feasibility trials 182
femoral (deep) inguinal lymphatics 30, 32, 33
femoral (Scarpa's) triangle 30
fine-needle aspiration biopsy (FNAB) 91
flow cytometry (FCM) 91–2
fluorescein 68
fossa ovalis 30
frozen section analysis 85–7, 159, 160

Galen 3
gamma detectors 75–6, 106, 163

Garcia, Ramiro 7
gluteal lymph nodes 44
Goddard, H. 2
Gould, E. 7
Gray, J. 3
groin
    anatomical illustrations 34–9, 35, 36, 37
        surgical compartments 38, 39
    embryology 27
    lymphatics
        deep 30, 32, 33
        superficial 30–2, 31
    topographic anatomy 29–30, 29, 31
Gynecologic Oncology Group (GOG) studies
        9–10, 79

Halsted model 3–5, 4, 18
history of lymphatic mapping 1–13
    cadaver studies 1–3, 2, 3
    Halsted model 3–5, 4, 18
    in vivo injection of dyes 5–7, 6
    progress toward modern concept 10–11
    SLN identification 7–10, 8
Hudack, Stephen 6
human papillomavirus (HPV) in cervix cancer
        125–6, 142–3
hysterectomy, radical 125, 128
hysteroscopy 175–6

Imferon 9
immunohistochemistry (IHC) 89–90, 89, 90
    breast cancer 90–1, 158, 159
    squamous cell carcinomas 91
immunology of regional lymph nodes 23
imprint cytology 87, 160
India ink injection 6
indigo carmine, absorbance spectrum 72
indoctamine green, absorbance spectrum 72
infiltrating lobular carcinoma, breast 149
inguinal lymphatics
    deep 30, 32, 33
    superficial 30–2, 31
inguinal nodes, Way illustration 5
inguinofemoral lymphadenectomy, vulvar cancer
        4, 9, 102–3, 118, 119
innovation, diffusion of 179–80
institutional review board approval 180–1
invasive duct carcinoma, breast 148

in vivo injection of dyes see blue dyes
isosulfan blue
    absorbance spectrum 72
    features 68
    molecular structure 68
    side effects 70–1, 72, 142, 160

Lancaster, John 179
laparoscopic SLN mapping, cervix cancer 140–2
Leveuf, J. 2
lobular carcinoma in situ, breast (LCIS) 148, 148
lymph 20
lymphadenectomy, lymphedema following 24,
        25
lymphatic capillaries 18, 19
lymphatic channels 1–2, 19
lymphatic system, anatomy and physiology
    early studies 1–3, 2, 3, 17
    lymph 20
    lymphatic vessels 18–19, 19
    lymph nodes see lymph nodes
    surgical anatomy 24
lymphedema 24, 25
lymph nodes
    anatomy 21
    antigen recognition 22
    immunology 23
    metastasis rates 22
    passage of lymph through 21
    second echelon 67, 74, 74, 75
    sentinal see sentinal lymph nodes (SLNs)
    surgical counts 24
    see also specific anatomical regions
lymphocysts 24
lymphography of the penis (Cabanas' technique)
        7, 8
lymphoscintigraphy (LSG) 72–8
    advantages 72
    applicability and availability 80
    delayed scans 74, 74
    efficacy 78–9
    gamma detectors 75–6, 106, 163
    introduction 10, 10
    lymph flow rate studies 20
    radiocolloids see radiocolloids
    safety
        patients 77–8
        staff 77

lymphoscintigraphy (LSG) *cont.*
    technique 74, 76–7
    see also specific cancers: SLN mapping entries

McMaster, Phillip 6
melanoma
    cutaneous
        and lymph node immune responses 23
        lymphoscintigraphy 10, *10*
        SLN procedure in 120
        suitability for lymphatic mapping *172*
    randomized clinical trials 184–5, *185*, *186*
    vulvar, SLN procedure in 118–19, *118*, *119*
methylene blue 68, 72
Morton, Donald 10–11
MUC1 90–1
Multicenter Selective Lymphadenectomy Trial
        120, 184–5, *185*

National Surgical Adjuvant Breast and Bowel
        Project (NSABP) B–32 trial 185–6, *187*
NCRC11 91
node counts 24

observational trial design 184
obturator lymph nodes 44
ovarian cancer
    lymph node metastases 56
    modes of dissemination 55
    SLN detection 57
ovaries, lymphatic anatomy 55, *57*

parametrial lymph nodes 43–4
Parry-Jones, E. 9
patent blue-V dye 68, 160
pathologists, radiation doses to 78
pathology *see* ultrastaging of SLNs
pectoralis muscles 59
pelvic lymphatics, early drawings *2*
pelvic lymph nodes
    metastases
        endometrial cancer 52–3
        ovarian cancer 56
    Way illustration *5*
penile lymphography, Cabanas' technique 7, *8*
positron emission tomography (PET), cervix
        cancer evaluation 126
posterior interiliac nodes 44

preclinical trials 182
pregnant staff, radiation safety 78
pulse oximetry, effects of blue dyes 71–2

QWERTY keyboard 179

radiation protection 77–8
radical hysterectomy 125, 128
radical vulvectomy 4, 9
radiocolloids
    compared *73*
    early use 10
    efficacy of lymphatic mapping with 78–9
    flow rates 73–4
    ideal characteristics 73
    injection technique 76
    safety
        patients 77–8
        staff 77
randomized clinical trials
    examples 184–8, *185*, *186*, *187*, *188*
    features 184
    gynecologic cancer 188
    statistical analysis 182
reverse-transcriptase polymerase chain reaction
        (RT-PCR) 92–3, 143
Riveros, Manuel 7
Rosenmüller's (Cloquet's) node 30, 32

safety
    blue dye methods 70–2, *72*, 142, 160
    lymphoscintigraphy 77–8
Scarpa's triangle 30
scintillation gamma detectors 75
semiconductor gamma detectors 75
sentinal lymph nodes (SLNs)
    definitions 67, *154*
    dendritic cell function 23
    detection modalities 67–83
    early efforts at identification 7–10, *8*, 11
    introduction of concept 1, 7, 9, 153
    mapping procedures *see specific cancers: SLN
        mapping entries*
    pathologic analysis *see* ultrastaging of SLNs
    radioactive, definitions *183*
    vs. second echelon nodes 67, 74, *74*, *75*
serial section analysis 88–9, *88*, *89*
Starling, E.H. 17

statistical analysis of clinical trials 181–2, *182*
sulfur microcolloid 20
Sunbelt Melanoma Trial 185, *186*
superficial inguinal lymphadenectomy 9, 10
superficial inguinal lymphatics 30–2, *31*
superficial perineal fascia 27, *28*
surgeons
   learning curves *122*, 161
   radiation exposure 78
surgery
   approaches to the groin 38, *39*
   cervix cancer 125, 128
   vulvar cancer 4, 9, 34
surgical anatomy of the lymphatic system 24

technetium(Tc)-labelled radiocolloids 73, *73*, 77–8
terminal lymphatics 18, *19*
thoracic duct 21, *22*
thorium oxide injections 17
transperitoneal lymphadenectomy, cervix cancer 131
tumor—node—metastasis (TNM) system 34
   breast cancer 149–52, *149–51*, *152*

ultrasonographically guided FNAB 91
ultrastaging of SLNs 85–100
   fine-needle aspiration cytology 91
   flow cytometry 91–2
   immunohistochemistry *see* immunohisto-
      chemistry (IHC)
   intraoperative
      frozen section analysis 85–7
      imprint cytology 87, 160
   optimal protocol determination 94–5
   recommendations *95*
   RT-PCR 92–3
   serial section analysis 88–9, *88*, *89*
urogenital diaphragm 27
urticaria, due to isosulfan blue 70

uterosacral ligaments 42, *42*
uterus *see* cervix; corpus uteri

validation trial design 182–3, *183*
Valsava, Antonio M. 3
vulva
   embryology 27
   lymphatic drainage 32, *38*
      Eichner's work 7
      Parry-Jones' observations 9
      Sappey illustration 2, *3*
   topographic anatomy 27, *28*
   see also groin
vulvar cancer
   natural history and spread 34, 101
   prognosis 101
   staging system *102*
   suitability for lymphatic mapping *172*
   surgical management 34, 102
vulvar cancer, SLN mapping 69, 79, 101–24
   clinical implementation 120, 121
   learning curve reduction *122*
   melanoma 118–19, *118*, *119*
   published studies 113–15, *116–17*, 184, 188
   rationale 101–3
   squamous cell carcinoma
      patient selection 103–4
      patient care before admission 104
      lymphoscintigraphy 104–6, *104*, *105*, *106*, *107*
      operative procedure 107–13, *108*, *109*, *110*, *111*, *112*, *113*
      frozen section analysis 110
      pathologic examination 113
vulvectomy, radical 4, 9

Way, Stanley 4–5, *5*

Xerox Corporation 179